More Praise for *Johns Hopkins Pat*

"Drs. Hesdorffer and Morrison have everyone who has been given the diagnosis of leukemia. They provide important information about this frightening disease in a clearly understandable and accessible manner. They use language which is simple and yet scientifically accurate. Anyone who has leukemia or whose loved one has leukemia will find this book most helpful in negotiating through the maze of tests and treatment choices and uncertainties of what might come next. All of us who treat patients with various forms of leukemia have long realized a dire need for just such a resource book and arrival of this book is most welcome.

We are grateful to Drs. Hesdorffer and Morrison for providing a most needed source of information on leukemia. This book is expertly written and explains very complex concepts in clear and understandable manner."

Kanti R. Rai, MD
Long Island Jewish Medical Center

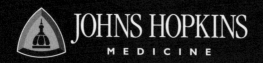
Patients' Guide to

Leukemia

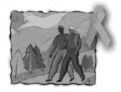

Candis Morrison, PhD, CRNP

Nurse Practitioner, Division of Hematology
Johns Hopkins Medical Institutions
Baltimore, MD

Charles S. Hesdorffer, MBBCh, MMED

Staff Clinician, National Institute on Aging PLSA/CRB
Harbor Hospital
Baltimore, MD

SERIES EDITORS
Lillie D. Shockney, RN, BS, MAS

University Distinguished Service Associate Professor of Breast Cancer; Administrative Director of Breast Cancer; Associate Professor, Department of Surgery; Associate Professor, Department of Obstetrics and Gynecology, Johns Hopkins School of Medicine; Associate Professor, Johns Hopkins School of Nursing

Gary R. Shapiro, MD

Chairman, Department of Oncology
Johns Hopkins Bayview Medical Center
Director, Johns Hopkins Geriatric Oncology Program
The Sidney Kimmel Comprehensive Cancer Center at Johns Hopkins

JONES & BARTLETT
L E A R N I N G

World Headquarters
Jones & Bartlett Learning
40 Tall Pine Drive
Sudbury, MA 01776
978-443-5000
info@jblearning.com
www.jblearning.com

Jones & Bartlett Learning
Canada
6339 Ormindale Way
Mississauga, Ontario L5V 1J2
Canada

Jones & Bartlett Learning
International
Barb House, Barb Mews
London W6 7PA
United Kingdom

Jones & Bartlett Learning books and products are available through most bookstores and online booksellers. To contact Jones & Bartlett Learning directly, call 800-832-0034, fax 978-443-8000, or visit our website, www.jblearning.com.

Substantial discounts on bulk quantities of Jones & Bartlett Learning publications are available to corporations, professional associations, and other qualified organizations. For details and specific discount information, contact the special sales department at Jones & Bartlett Learning via the above contact information or send an email to specialsales@jblearning.com.

The authors, editor, and publisher have made every effort to provide accurate information. However, they are not responsible for errors, omissions, or for any outcomes related to the use of the contents of this book and take no responsibility for the use of the products and procedures described. Treatments and side effects described in this book may not be applicable to all people; likewise, some people may require a dose or experience a side effect that is not described herein. Drugs and medical devices are discussed that may have limited availability controlled by the Food and Drug Administration (FDA) for use only in a research study or clinical trial. Research, clinical practice, and government regulations often change the accepted standard in this field. When consideration is being given to use of any drug in the clinical setting, the healthcare provider or reader is responsible for determining FDA status of the drug, reading the package insert, and reviewing prescribing information for the most up-to-date recommendations on dose, precautions, and contraindications, and determining the appropriate usage for the product. This is especially important in the case of drugs that are new or seldom used.

Production Credits
Executive Publisher: Christopher Davis
Editorial Assistant: Sara Cameron
Associate Production Editor: Laura Almozara
Associate Marketing Manager: Katie Hennessy
V.P., Manufacturing and Inventory Control: Therese Connell
Composition: Appingo Publishing Services
Cover Design: Kristin E. Parker
Cover Image: © ImageZoo/age fotostock
Printing and Binding: Malloy, Inc.
Cover Printing: Malloy, Inc.

Library of Congress Cataloging-in-Publication Data
Morrison, Candis.
    Johns Hopkins patients' guide to leukemia / Candis Morrison, Charles S. Hesdorffer.
      p. cm.
    Includes index.
    ISBN-13: 978-0-7637-7433-2
    ISBN-10: 0-7637-7433-2
    1. Leukemia—Popular works. I. Hesdorffer, Charles S. II. Title. III. Title: Patients' guide to leukemia.
    RC643.M66 2011
    616.99'419—dc22
                                                        2010010690

6048

Printed in the United States of America
14 13 12 11 10   10 9 8 7 6 5 4 3 2 1

DEDICATION

This book is dedicated to leukemia patients, their families, and friends, as well as to the teams of healthcare professionals that dedicate their careers and their hearts to improving the survival and the quality of life for patients with leukemia.

A special dedication is offered to the memory of Dr. Martin D. Ableoff, the Director of the Sidney Kimmel Comprehensive Cancer Center at Johns Hopkins from 1992 to 2007, and also a leukemia patient. We are grateful for his steadfast dedication to patient care and for his skillful leadership that allowed our cancer center to grow and thrive, becoming a Center for Excellence for many types of cancer.

Contents

Preface

Receiving a diagnosis of leukemia is a frightening experience. The term leukemia provokes scary images and a great deal of uncertainty about the future. Hearing the diagnosis was most likely a shock, especially if you were feeling relatively well prior to being told that you have this disease.

Knowledge about the disease and the healthcare system that treats patients with leukemia will help you cope with the diagnosis and all of its implications and better deal with your treatment. The good news is that there are more treatment choices now than ever before and survival rates have improved dramatically thanks to the research that has been conducted over the course of the past several decades.

The purposes of this book are to arm you with the information that you need to help you become an active participant in your care team and to inform your decisions regarding your treatment. It is meant as a guide and supplement for you and your family.

This book is part of a series of *Johns Hopkins Cancer Patient Guides* designed to educate newly diagnosed patients about their cancer diagnosis and the treatments that may lie ahead.

Please do not feel the need to read the entire book at once. It is intended for you to read at your leisure and when you feel ready to absorb additional information. It will supplement what you learn from your doctors and nurses. Additional resources for you are listed in Chapter 11.

Candis Morrison, PhD, CRNP

Charles S. Hesdorffer, MBBCh, MMED

Introduction

How to Use This Book
to Your Benefit

After you are informed that you have leukemia, you will begin to receive a great deal of information. This will come from your healthcare team, your family, and your friends. You will likely search the Internet, turning your computer off with more questions in mind than when you turned it on. Family and friends will want to provide advice on where to go and what to do.

Since leukemia is actually a group of many diseases, each with very different treatments and outcomes, it is crucial that you get specific information from the professionals in whom you have entrusted your care. Your situation is very likely different from those individuals you may hear about from well-meaning family members, friends, and coworkers. This book will help you understand the different types of leukemia and explain how they are treated. It is broken down into chapters with a list of additional resources including trustworthy Web sites to help empower you with accurate and understandable information. This will hopefully help get you on track to participate in the best plan of care for your leukemia.

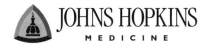

FIRST STEPS—
I'VE BEEN DIAGNOSED WITH
LEUKEMIA

R eceiving the diagnosis of leukemia is actually the first stage of your journey to recovery. It began with the first sign, symptom, or blood test that provoked concern. The thoughts, suspicions, and fears that followed have become a reality that requires our organized plan of attack.

Many patients are initially immobilized by the shock that came after the diagnosis. Others mobilize immediately, though not in a focused and constructive manner. In this book, we will start at the beginning of the journey with the goal of helping you and your family move smoothly through the stages of diagnosis confirmation, treatment, and post-treatment.

SELECTING YOUR ONCOLOGIST
AND MEDICAL CENTER

You will want to be in the hands of experts; this isn't a simple gallbladder problem or hernia repair, this is cancer! Don't rely on self-promoting advertisements on television as your way to select a facility and doctor. Your personal physician may be able to point you toward the best oncologists and the best cancer centers in your area. Major cancer centers are designated by the National Cancer Institute as part of the National Comprehensive Cancer Network, and are good sources for your care or for second opinions. This designation ensures that the center has met certain scientific, organizational, and administrative standards.

Leukemia is a disorder that requires a specialized staff and a multidisciplinary healthcare team that is dedicated to providing the most current state-of-the-art treatment and the support that the leukemia patient (and his or her family) needs from diagnosis to cure. If you are not currently being treated in such a facility, your doctor may refer you to one. Just as surgeons may specialize in orthopedics, vascular conditions, or neurological conditions, leukemia doctors can specialize in one or more of the different types of leukemia. This specialization means that the doctors and their teams are aware of the most current treatment strategies and have the most experience providing them to patients. This helps improve outcomes. They may also be able to offer new or different combinations of medicines on clinical trials that have been designed in an effort to improve the standards of care for your disease.

It is often advisable to get a second opinion after an initial consultation, particularly if the provider or facility does not have expertise in leukemia management. Insurance companies generally encourage an opinion from another specialist to ensure that you are being offered the best possible treatment. If time permits, this is a good idea. You also need to be comfortable with your doctor and the staff that will assist in your care.

While it is not wrong to shop around until you find an office or program that meets your needs based on location, expertise, and the compassion that you sense in the providers, be careful not to get too many opinions as it will likely confuse you and waste crucial time as well. Further resources are listed in Chapter 11.

GATHERING RECORDS: BIOPSY, LABS, AND RADIOLOGY REPORTS

As soon as you hear the words, "You have leukemia," request a copy of your laboratory reports, scans, and the pathology report if you have undergone bone marrow or lymph node biopsy. Be sure to obtain copies of all your medical records and continue to request copies as you continue through this journey so you maintain your own portfolio of treatments and test results. Although a report of the findings is helpful, your oncologist will want to review the actual films or images taken, and in the case of pathology, it is important to have the actual pathology slides sent to your treating facility to be reviewed by its pathologists. Find out from the referring facility how to get these materials to your oncologist. It may be best for you to pick them up and hand-carry them with you to your first consultation visit.

You may wonder why you need to get these films and slides if the reports have been made available. Accredited cancer centers and consultants will review the images and, most importantly, examine the pathology slides to verify their accuracy. Your treatment outcome is dependent on the accuracy of the diagnosis.

Consider starting a notebook or binder. This can serve as a journal that you can use to record visits, treatments, any side effects of medications or other important symptoms (such as fever), and consultations. This will also provide you with a place to keep business cards, comments, and contact information for those on your leukemia care team. These journals can come in handy to accurately relay important information regarding what is happening with you at each point during the process. Information provided, particularly during early visits that can be extremely stressful, is likely to seem overwhelming. Most people can only absorb about 50% of what they are told even when they are not stressed or upset. In addition, as time goes by, it is easy to confuse events and dates. It is therefore very helpful to have this information to refer back to for clarification.

LEARNING ABOUT YOUR DISEASE BEFORE THE FIRST VISIT

The term leukemia comes from a Greek work that means white blood. The leukemias are a group of malignant blood disorders that affect the immature blood-forming cells in the bone marrow. They are cancers of the blood and have actually been called "liquid tumors," while diseases such as breast, lung, and colon cancer are called "solid tumors." To better understand leukemia, it is helpful to know where and how normal blood cells develop and what their functions are in the body.

NORMAL DEVELOPMENT OF BLOOD CELLS

Blood cells are formed in the bone marrow, which is, in a sense, a factory for blood. There is marrow within many bones throughout the body, including the pelvis, some long bones, the skull, the breast bone, and the ribs. The bone marrow supports stem cells that are the most basic and primitive form of blood cells from which all other blood cells originate. Stem cells do not circulate in the blood, but each will differentiate (mature) into a white blood cell (WBC), red blood cell (RBC), or platelet in the marrow. They will eventually be released from the marrow into the peripheral circulation in an even more mature form based on the needs of the body at that particular time (Figure 1).

RBCs (also called erythrocytes) pick up oxygen from the lungs and carry it to tissues throughout the body in the form of hemoglobin. They also remove carbon dioxide, which is the waste product of breathing. Hematocrit is the term for the percentage of RBCs in the blood. In a healthy woman, the hematocrit ranges from 36%–46%. In men, the range is slightly higher at 40%–52%. Under normal

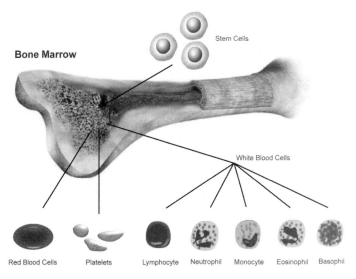

Figure 1 Bone marrow components.

conditions, the marrow produces enough RBCs to meet the needs of the body. When there is not enough hemoglobin, the patient is said to have anemia. Mild anemia is associated with a hematocrit from 30% to 35%, moderate anemia between 25% and 30%, and severe anemia is diagnosed when the hematocrit is 25% or less. At this point, patients may require RBC transfusions. Anemia may cause fatigue, weakness, palpitations, shortness of breath, dizziness, and even chest pain. Anemic patients may appear pale and may have a rapid heart rate.

Platelets, also called thrombocytes, are the smallest of the blood cells. They work by clumping together to form clots and thus prevent bleeding. Healthy marrow generally insures that there are between 150,000 and 450,000 platelets per microliter of blood. Severe bleeding rarely occurs unless the platelet count drops below 10,000. When there are too few platelets in the blood, the patient also bruises easily and may have nosebleeds and/or bleeding from the gums, stomach, or bowels. Pinpoint bruises under the skin, called petechiae, are also associated with low platelet counts.

WBCs, or leukocytes, protect the body from infections. There are two major types of WBCs: neutrophils (also called granulocytes or polys) fight bacterial infections, while lymphocytes fight viral infections and produce antibodies to protect from past infections such as measles or mumps. Other types of WBCs are counted in a test called the differential. These are fewer in number and include monocytes, eosinophils, and basophils. When WBCs are too low, the immune system is not able to do its job as effectively and you are more likely to become ill. Fever and chills are generally the first signs of infection as the immune system tries to "rev up" to protect you from invading organisms.

The body produces special messengers to tell the stem cells which type of cell is needed at any particular time. For example, if you have a bacterial infection, a messenger substance is released that will stimulate the bone marrow to produce neutrophils. If you cut yourself and lose a great deal of blood, there is another messenger released by the kidneys (when they sense the decrease in your blood volume), and the stem cells mature into RBCs so that you do not become too anemic.

Based on the message they receive, stem cells differentiate into slightly more mature cells blasts. Blasts normally reside in the bone marrow and do not circulate in the peripheral blood; rather they continue to mature prior to being released into peripheral blood circulation. These cells then circulate in the body, performing their respective jobs until they grow old, or become damaged, and then die in a genetically predetermined period of time. This process of programmed cell death is called apoptosis. In this way, the rate of blood cell production varies according to the needs of the body. Old cells die and are replaced by new ones in an organized process (Figure 2).

WHAT ARE THE TYPES OF LEUKEMIA?

There are several types of leukemia. They are grouped both by the type of cells (lymphoid or myeloid) that are abnormal, and by the rate of abnormal cell growth. When leukemia develops, the normal maturation process is disrupted and one, or both, of two major problems may occur.

Acute Leukemias

The first problem is one in which cell maturity is disrupted, resulting in increasing numbers of very immature cells

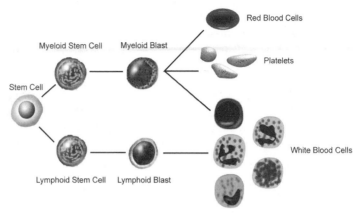

Figure 2 This diagram pictures how stem cells mature into the type of cell needed by the body at a given time. The lymphoid stem cell first becomes a lymphoid blast that can mature into either a B or T lymphocyte. A myeloid stem cell first becomes a myeloid blast which can then mature into a red blood cell, a platelet, or one of several types of non-lymphoid white blood cells (neutrophil, basophil, eosinophil, or monocyte).

(the blasts) in the marrow and in the circulation. Remember that under normal conditions, blasts are not seen in the peripheral blood but they are in cases of acute leukemias.

Acute leukemias can be life-threatening because there are not enough mature blood cells to fight infection and/or to prevent bleeding and severe anemia. Acute leukemia is diagnosed when there are 10% or more blasts in the bone marrow. Under normal conditions, there are 2% or less blasts in the marrow. The two most common acute leukemias are acute lymphocytic leukemia (ALL), and acute myeloid leukemia (AML). These differ based on the cell affected, the former from the lymphoid cell line and the latter from the myeloid line. These acute forms of leukemia are severe and aggressive. Blast cells can accumulate in the blood, bone marrow, organs, and possibly in the CNS.

Overproduction of the abnormal cells prevents growth of normal cells and results in low RBCs, platelets, and infection-fighting WBCs.

Chronic Leukemias

The second major defect leading to leukemia involves mature WBCs that don't die off in that normally organized fashion, known as apoptosis. Cells, therefore, continue to accumulate in the circulation and bone marrow and can cause marrow crowding that can disrupt production of other cell lines that are otherwise normal. They may also accumulate in the lymph nodes and spleen, causing them to increase in size. This is typical of the chronic leukemias.

Chronic leukemias generally progress slowly and patients may not have any symptoms for years. They are often diagnosed during evaluation for another problem, or during laboratory studies for a routine physical exam. As the disease progresses, lymph nodes may become more enlarged, though this is generally painless enlargement. The patient may also experience more frequent infections. The two most common chronic leukemias are chronic lymphocytic leukemia (CLL) and chronic myelogenous leukemia (CML). These also differ based on the cell affected, the former from the lymphoid cell line and the latter from the myeloid line.

Myelodysplastic Syndrome

In addition to acute and chronic leukemia, there is a condition called myelodysplastic syndrome (MDS), which is actually a group of diseases in which there is an insufficient production of normal bone marrow and blood cells. The bone marrow becomes unable to make enough normal blood cells to sustain the needs of the body. Patients may have low numbers of WBCs, RBCs, and/or platelets and may need RBC and/or platelet transfusions. Some patients with MDS develop acute leukemia over time.

MDS is diagnosed by evaluation of the bone marrow. This test is generally recommended after doctors find low cell counts on the complete blood count (CBC).

See Table 1 for a list of some of the leukemias. Each of the major leukemias will be discussed in more detail later in this chapter and in Chapter 3.

WHAT ARE THE SYMPTOMS OF LEUKEMIA?

Symptoms of leukemia generally include fatigue and weakness. These may develop slowly, or very rapidly, depending on the type of leukemia. Patients may look pale and lose weight unintentionally. They may have fevers, drenching night sweats, and a loss of appetite, and they may get frequent, and/or severe infections. Bruising may occur and patients may bleed easily, experiencing nosebleeds or bleeding from their gums when they brush their teeth. Patients with acute leukemia are generally very ill when they present for evaluation and treatment. Lymph nodes may become swollen and may be painful. Patients may also complain of bone or joint pain and may have tenderness in the upper abdomen caused by a swollen liver or spleen.

Alternatively, chronic leukemia may not have any symptoms and may be diagnosed incidentally during evaluation for another problem or during a routine physical exam for an unrelated reason. Patients may experience some of the symptoms that those with acute leukemia develop, though they are generally much less severe.

Table 1 Leukemias

Acute Leukemias	Chronic Leukemias	Myelodysplastic Syndromes
Acute Lymphoblastic Leukemia (ALL) • T-cell ALL • B-cell ALL (including Burkitt's leukemia/ lymphoma) • Lymphoblastic lymphoma	Chronic Lymphocytic Leukemia (CLL) • Mantle zone leukemia • Marginal zone leukemia • Hairy cell leukemia • Splenic lymphoma	Myelodysplastic Syndromes (MSDs) • Refractory anemias • Chronic myelo-monocytic leukemia
Acute Myelogenous Leukemia (AML) • Acute myelomono-cytic leukemia • Acute monocytic leukemia • Acute promyelo-cytic leukemia • Acute erythroleukemia • Acute megakaryo-cytic leukemia	Chronic Myelogenous Leukemia (CML)	
Acute Undifferentiated Leukemia	Myeloproliferative Syndromes • Myelofibrosis • Polycythemia vera • Essential thrombo-cytosis	

HOW COMMON IS LEUKEMIA?

Almost 45,000 individuals are diagnosed with leukemia each year in the United States. When the 16 most common separate cancer sites were compared, leukemia was the 12th most common class of neoplastic disease and the 11th most common cause of cancer-related death. In the United States, an estimated 5,500 cases of ALL and 13,000 cases of AML are diagnosed each year. CLL is the most common human leukemia with approximately 15,000 new cases each year and 86,000 people live with this disease. CML accounts for about 5,000 new leukemia diagnoses yearly. There are 12,000 new cases of MDS diagnosed each year and 55,000 patients are living with this disease.

Though leukemia is generally thought of as a childhood disease, it is diagnosed 10 times more frequently in adults than in children. In children up to 19 years of age, ALL is the most common form (72% of cases) of the disease. In adults, the most common leukemias are CLL and AML.

WHAT CAUSES LEUKEMIA?

The cause of leukemia for any given patient is usually not known and cannot be identified. There are, however, identifiable cellular changes that occur. Leukemia, like other cancers, begins with a mutation in the genetic material within cells. Every cell in your body has the same DNA, which is the genetic material that is inherited from your parents. The DNA contains the genes that control the activity of the cell. DNA is copied into new cells each time they divide and during this division, there is the opportunity for errors in replication to occur. These errors may lead to the creation of leukemia cells instead of normal cells.

Several risk factors have been linked to development of leukemia, though it is uncertain why some individuals with these factors develop the disease and others do not.

Identified risk factors include:

Male gender. Leukemia is more common in males than in females.

Older age. Approximately 60%–70% of leukemias occur in individuals over the age of 50.

Genetic syndromes. Individuals with Downs syndrome have a 15-fold increase in the risk of developing leukemia. Other inherited disorders associated with increased risk are Ataxia Telangiectasia, Fanconi anemia, and Bloom syndrome.

Exposure to radiation. The risk of developing several forms of leukemia is increased in individuals who were exposed to high doses of radiation. Examples include the people that were exposed to the radiation released during the atomic bombing in Japan in World War II, military personnel involved in nuclear testing in the 1950s, and those exposed to the Chernobyl reactor accident in Russia. X-rays used for routine diagnostic purposes are not thought to pose risk.

Racial and ethnic factors. Rates of CLL are higher in some Jewish populations while it is rare in Asians.

Family history. There is a two- to four-fold increase in risk for CLL in first-degree relatives of CLL patients.

Chemical exposure. Workers exposed to the chemical benzene have a 20-fold increased risk of developing leukemia (AML, CML, or ALL). Benzene is found in some solvents, herbicides, and pesticides. It is also present in cigarette smoke, putting smokers and secondhand smokers at increased risk. Other chemicals that may increase risk include ethylene oxides, dioxin, butadienes, and styrenes.

Medications. Childhood leukemia has been linked to the use of the antibiotic Chloromycetin (chloramphenicol). Growth hormones and Butazolidin (phenylbutazone) have also been suspected causative factors. Immunosuppressive agents such as those used after organ transplantation to prevent rejection have been linked to the development of some leukemias and lymphomas.

Viral factors. Development of acute T-cell leukemia has been linked to the human T-cell leukemia virus I (HTLV-I). This association is more common in Asia and the Caribbean than it is in the United States. Some animal viruses have been implicated in butchers and in veterinary staff who develop leukemia.

History of cancer therapy. Those who have received chemotherapy and radiation for prior cancers are at a slightly higher risk of developing AML than the general population. The highest risk chemotherapy agents are those used in the treatment of breast and ovarian cancers, as well as blood malignancies such as Hodgkin's disease. Implicated chemotherapeutics include, but are not limited to, Cytoxan (cyclophosphamide), Leukeran (chlorambucil), Etopophos (etoposide), and Mustargen (mechlorethamine). Radiation therapy used in conjunction with chemotherapy increases the risk.

CAN LEUKEMIA BE PREVENTED?

Risk factors such as age, gender, and ethnicity obviously cannot be modified. Avoiding cigarette smoke and other known chemicals linked to the development of leukemia is the only known way to modify one's risk. Early detection of leukemia is also difficult because the symptoms are generally vague and may thus be attributed to other causes until the appropriate blood tests are performed.

LEUKEMIA STAGING

Leukemia is staged differently than are solid tumors. You may be familiar with the common cancer terminology of Stages I through IV that is used for lung, breast, and other common tumors. The term stage connotes how much disease is present in the body (how many body areas are affected). Since leukemia is a cancer of the blood and or lymphatic systems, it is more likely to be in the bone marrow, the lymph nodes, the liver, and the spleen when it is first diagnosed.

CHRONIC LEUKEMIA STAGING

Chronic Lymphocytic Leukemia

There are two different staging systems for CLL. In the United States, the Rai classification is most commonly used. Rai stages range from 0 to IV and are correlated with assessment of risk. While Stage 0 is deemed low risk, Stages I and II are intermediate, and III and IV are high risk. In Rai stage 0, the only abnormality is a high lymphocyte count (generally over 15,000 lymphocytes per cubic millimeter). There are no symptoms and the other blood counts are completely normal. An increased number of lymphocytes is called lymphocytosis.

In Rai Stage I, the patient has enlarged lymph nodes (called lympadenopathy) as well as lymphocytosis. Rai Stage II consists of lymphocytosis as well as an enlarged liver or spleen. In this stage, lympadenopathy may or may not be present.

Rai Stage III consists of lymphocytosis and anemia, with or without lymphadenopathy, and with or without an enlarged liver and/or spleen. In Rai Stage IV, the patient has lymphocytosis and low platelet count (thrombocytopenia). This is the most advanced stage of CLL.

The Binet staging system, which is more widely used in Europe, for CLL consists of three stages (A through C). In Stage A, there are fewer than three areas of enlarged lymphoid tissue, while in B there are more than three. In Binet Stage C, the patient has anemia and thromobocytopenia.

Chronic Myelogeneous Leukemia

CML is characterized by specific chromosomal changes and the observance of the Philadelphia Chromosome, which is the marker for CML, when the leukemia cells are analyzed. The Philadelphia Chromosome contains an abnormal gene called the BCR-ABL gene that causes the body to make too many WBCs. CML is divided into three phases (the term phase is used instead of stage when referring to CML).

In chronic phase CML, there are less than 5% blasts in the blood and marrow samples. In this stage there are few, or mild, symptoms, and they generally respond readily to therapy.

The second phase is the accelerated phase in which bone marrow and blood samples contain between 5% and 30% blasts. Symptoms at this stage may include poor appetite, weight loss, and fever. In this phase, the disease is less responsive to treatment

The final phase is the acute phase, or the blast phase or blast crisis. In this phase, there are greater than 30% blasts. Anemia and infections are common in patients in blast phase.

Blood tests with cytogenetic analysis are performed to confirm and quantify the current disease status. Fluorescence in situ hybridization (FISH) measures the percentage of CML cells. Polymerase chain reaction (PCR) is used when there is a smaller quantity of CML cells than FISH can detect. These tests are also conducted during chemotherapy to monitor its effectiveness. Fortunately, they can be performed using peripheral blood now. In the past, repeated bone marrow examinations were required.

ACUTE LEUKEMIA STAGING

Acute Lymphocytic Leukemia and Acute Mylogenous Leukemia

There are no standard staging systems for ALL or AML. In adults, ALL is classified as untreated, in remission, or recurrent. In children, risk groups are used to describe the disease and include standard risk (low risk), high risk, or recurrent.

MYELODYSPASTIC SYNDROME STAGING

Since there is a great deal of variation in disease course, MDS risk groups have been developed to help classify them. This system is called the International Prognostic Scoring System (IPSS). It is based on findings from the physical examination and lab tests, including the percentage of blasts in the marrow, the cytogenetic findings in the marrow cells, and the blood counts (see page 22 for more information). The score reflects chances of progression to acute leukemia and thus can be used to estimate life expectancy. Risk groups include low risk (score of 0), intermediate 1 risk (score of 0.5–1.0), intermediate 2 risk (score of 1.5–2.0), and high risk (over 2.0).

SUMMARY

This information has hopefully given you a better understanding of leukemia and MDS, but it has probably also provoked a number of questions. Please bring these questions to the attention of your healthcare team. Chapter 3 of this book will discuss particular treatment aspects of each type of leukemia and Chapter 11 provides additional educational resources and Web sites for you to consult during your journey.

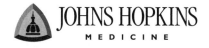

CHAPTER 2

MY TEAM—
MEETING YOUR
TREATMENT TEAM

YOUR HEALTHCARE TEAM

There will be many members of your leukemia care team. Each has a specific role and area of specialty and will contribute his or her expertise during your care. The following is a list of the major members of your team with a brief description of their roles:

Medical oncologist or hematologist. This specialist will be the leader of your team. This is the doctor that will complete your diagnostic evaluation and develop your plan of care, including any chemotherapy or antibody therapy that is required. You will see this doctor as an outpatient and if you are admitted to the hospital, the doctor will follow you through the hospitalization.

Radiation oncologist. If consulted in your care, this doctor will design and deliver radiation to help cure or control your disease. This therapy is delivered in a Radiation Oncology Center.

Surgeon. Various surgeons may be enlisted to assist in your care. For instance, if you need a biopsy of a lymph node to help make the diagnosis, or if you need an intravenous catheter placed through which your chemotherapy can be delivered, a surgeon will perform these procedures.

Pathologist. The pathologist views tissue and blood under a microscope. He or she helps diagnose your leukemia by looking at the lymph nodes, blood, and bone marrow.

Nurse practitioner (NP). NPs are advanced practice nurses who are educated in a particular field of practice. They can help you in many of the same ways that your doctors do. Your NP will help you to manage your symptoms, care for you during treatment, write your prescriptions, and order lab tests.

Physician assistant. Physician assistants help doctors care for you in the same manner as NPs. They may be involved in your diagnosis and/or treatment, as well as during follow-up visits to the clinic after your treatment.

Registered nurses. Nurses who have special education in the areas of hematology and oncology will help care for you, too. They are responsible for conducting assessments and will provide your therapy. They will teach you about your disease, your specific treatment's common side effects, and how you can best care for yourself during treatment.

Research nurses. If you are eligible for a clinical trial, a research nurse will discuss this with you and assess your desire to participate. If you choose to participate, this nurse will follow you along with your doctors and other nurses throughout your treatment.

Social Worker. This is someone who specializes in support during and after your diagnosis and will help in addressing any financial issues related to your care. The social worker can also help you access particular organizations that can help you as well.

Survivor Volunteer. There may be access to individuals who have had leukemia and have chosen to volunteer in the Center by providing one-on-one support to newly diagnosed leukemia patients. This individual is able to provide a candid view of what to expect and can be a great source of support along your journey.

The individuals on your treatment team will share information regarding your status on a frequent basis. You will receive their contact information and instructions regarding how to best reach them.

QUESTIONS TO ASK DURING YOUR INITIAL APPOINTMENT

After you have selected your treatment team and scheduled your initial appointment, it is helpful to prepare a list of questions to ask your doctor. The following is a list to help get you started:

1. Exactly what type of leukemia do I have?

2. How soon should my therapy begin?

3. How long has this center been treating patients with my condition?

4. Will there be nurses, case managers, and social workers available to help me with medical insurance and quality of life issues?

5. What are the therapy options for my disease?

6. Are there any clinical trials open in this center that I may be eligible for?

7. How long will my treatment last?

8. Who will manage my symptoms during therapy?

9. Who do I call if I do not feel well?

WHAT TESTS NEED TO BE DONE?

As discussed in the previous chapter, leukemia may be diagnosed during blood tests for a routine physical exam or for another reason. It may also be discovered during the evaluation of one of the symptoms mentioned in Chapter 1. A detailed history and physical examination is performed soon after diagnosis. It is important to have an accurate assessment of your health status including all past medical illnesses and surgeries, and to identify the effects of the recently diagnosed leukemia. Family history is important, especially since the health of your siblings may determine if they can provide bone marrow should you need a bone marrow/stem cell transplant at some point in the disease process. Some or all of the following blood tests will be ordered:

> *Complete blood count (CBC).* The CBC is used to assess the numbers of WBCs, RBCs, and platelets. A differential will be performed to determine the relative number and percentages of the different types of WBCs.

A smear of the peripheral blood. The blood smear can diagnose acute leukemia by demonstrating blasts. Bone marrow examination is required to characterize the leukemia.

Chemistry studies. Chemistry studies will be done to assess the function of the kidneys and the liver. This also provides information about blood sugar and electrolytes, such as sodium, potassium, and calcium.

Cardiac tests. An echocardiogram or multiple-gated acquisition scan (MUGA) may be arranged to get a baseline record of your heart's structure and function. Some of the agents used to treat leukemia (particularly an IV medication called Adriamycin [doxorubicin]) can affect the pumping action of the heart.

Lymph node biopsy. This is a relatively simple out-patient procedure during which a lymph node is removed entirely, in part, or aspirated using a needle and syringe. Lymph node excisions are performed by a surgeon. Sometimes a needle biopsy (FNA, or fine needle aspiration) will suffice, especially when the lymph nodes are in hard to reach places. This involves inserting a fine needle into the lymph node and removing cellular tissue (cytology) for examination in the pathology laboratory. If possible, a core biopsy is performed as it provides more tissue with more intact architecture. This type of biopsy may be performed under ultrasound or computed tomography guidance, and if so a radiologist will perform the procedure. It involves removing a small piece of the lymph node by inserting a larger biopsy needle into it. Lymph node biopsies are done to allow the pathologist to examine the leukemia cells under the microscope to help determine the specific type of leukemia you have.

Bone marrow biopsy and aspiration. This procedure, as the name suggests, requires inserting a small biopsy needle through the bone into the bone marrow (space in the bone involved in the production of blood cells). The biopsy site is usually in the back of your hipbone. The biopsy is usually done as an outpatient in your hematologist/oncologist's office to determine both the type of leukemia that you have as well as how much of your bone marrow has been replaced by the leukemia. It also provides material for cytogenetic analysis and immunophenotyping.

- *Cytogenetic analysis.* A look at the chromosomes in the cells that helps to better characterize the leukemia. These studies may be able to provide information regarding how the leukemia is expected to respond to therapy. Cytogenetics tests can also be performed on peripheral blood; however, different information is available from the marrow.

- *Immunophenotyping.* Also called flow cytometry, helps the pathologist establish the exact subtype of leukemia that is present. It determines which surface markers are on the leukemia cells. Different leukemias express different patterns of surface marker expression.

This procedure is crucial in the determination regarding most effective therapeutic options. Although you may experience some discomfort with the procedure, most people are able to tolerate the procedure well with generous amounts of local anesthesia. However, if you are worried about pain or if you had a bad experience with a previous bone marrow biopsy, the procedure could be done under sedation and you should speak to your physician about it.

Accurate diagnosis, prognosis, and management depend on this type of sophisticated testing. Because the diagnosis of leukemia, particularly its sub-types, can be difficult to make, it is important to have a pathologist with expertise in the diagnosis of leukemia review the biopsy material and the special tests results.

Spinal tap. A lumbar puncture or spinal tap may be required particularly in cases of acute leukemia to determine if the spinal fluid contains leukemia cells. For this procedure, the skin over the lower back is numbed with local anesthesia and a long thin needle is inserted into the space around the spinal cord. A small sample of spinal fluid is slowly removed with a syringe. In some acute leukemias, chemotherapy may be inserted during the same procedure to treat leukemia in the spinal fluid or to decrease the risk of the disease spreading to this area.

Radiographic studies. These may include:

* *X-rays or computed tomography (CAT) scans.* These are sometimes performed to evaluate for enlarged internal lymph nodes or organs that could be involved in leukemia. This may be part of the staging process to determine the extent of disease. CAT scans take multiple pictures as the camera rotates around the body. CAT produces cross-sectional pictures, or slices, that afford a great deal of detail about the anatomy of the organs and is capable of visualizing lymph nodes that cannot be palpated on physical examination. It is generally done with oral and intravenous contrast (dye) that better outlines the structures.

- *Magnetic resonance imaging (MRI) scans.* These use radiowaves and strong magnets instead of X-rays. They can produce detailed images of parts of the body and are especially useful for examining the spinal cord and the brain.

- *Positron emission tomography (PET) scans.* These may be ordered as well. In this study, a glucose-containing solution is injected with a radioactive atom prior to the scan. The glucose is then absorbed by areas that are metabolically active (e.g., cancers, inflammation). A special camera detects the radioactivity and produces a picture of the body. It has the ability to "light up" areas of the body that are involved with the disease and is a very sensitive imaging study.

Any, or all, of these studies may be repeated during and after therapy to insure that the chosen treatment is effective.

HOW TO BEST CONTACT TEAM MEMBERS

When you meet the members of your leukemia care team, it is a good idea to ask them how to contact them if you were to have problems or concerns. Some healthcare providers prefer to communicate by office phone, while others respond best by email. Keep any business or appointment cards that are given to you. These will provide contact numbers.

All doctors and cancer centers have emergency call numbers for you to use at night and on weekends in case serious problems arise. Be sure that you understand your team's policy for this coverage, and what information you need to have on hand when you call. For example, if you are not feeling well, take your temperature before your call. The on-call doctor will need this information. He or she may not have your medical records at the time of the call. Tell the doctor what type of leukemia you have, what treatment regimen you are on, and the date that you last received it. You should have a list or at least a thorough understanding of what is considered urgent or emergent and who to call when.

NAVIGATING APPOINTMENTS

Some cancer centers have patient navigators who help you with scheduling your evaluation and to navigate the healthcare system. These individuals may also be called patient care coordinators. Their purpose is to assist you in dealing with what can seem like an overwhelmingly complex system in which you may otherwise not know where to start.

If no such individual is available, inquire about who will help with scheduling and appointments issues. Who will assist with getting test results back and making sure that your consultations are conducted in a timely fashion? You need a clear understanding of what needs to occur when and who you need to contact to insure that it happens.

FINANCIAL IMPLICATIONS OF TREATMENT/ INSURANCE CLEARANCE

Many leukemia treatments will require some time away from work and your normal activities. Generally, the more acute the leukemia, the more intensive your therapy will be. Once you have a good understanding of what your treatment will involve and its estimated schedule, it is helpful to address the financial implications as early in the process as possible.

If you work outside of your home, find out about sick leave, short or long-term disability coverage benefits, prescription coverage, and copayment issues. For example, what is the visit and prescription copayment for which you are responsible? This is important to know prior to treatment so that you and your healthcare providers are aware of any limitations in your coverage. Another important question is whether you can have blood tests performed in the cancer center or whether you need to go to an outside lab. The same holds true for X-rays and scans—some insurers insist on using specific facilities, even though this may not be as convenient for you or your doctors.

If you choose to enter a clinical research study, the research nurse will help you determine what expenses will covered by your insurance company, and what expenses are covered under the study. Investigational drugs are generally supplied to you at no charge. Costs that are only study related and not considered standard of care should be paid for by the study. Neither you nor your insurance company is then responsible. There are very strict federal guidelines about these issues.

The fees for some services are bundled by insurance companies and cancer centers. Bone marrow/stem cell transplants are one example. This may also impact charges to your insurer and copayments for you. You should know about this up front.

If you do not have health insurance, it is crucial that you meet with financial counselors and/or your social worker as soon as possible. Facilities may not schedule services without financial clearance.

There are leukemia organizations and associations that may be able to help with some of the expenses that are not covered by your healthcare insurance. Your social worker is the best resource for their contact information; however, some of these resources are also listed in Chapter 11.

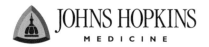

CHAPTER 3

TAKING ACTION— COMPREHENSIVE TREATMENT CONSIDERATIONS

Treatment for leukemia depends on the specific type and extent of the disease. Other important considerations include your age, general health status, and goals of the therapy. Therapy may include chemotherapy, radiation therapy, biologic therapy, surgery, and bone marrow/stem cell transplant. Depending on the exact type of leukemia, there may be other options, especially if the leukemia is chronic.

THERAPEUTIC MODALITIES

CHEMOTHERAPY

Treatment may consist of one or more chemotherapy drugs. These are delivered in cycles—the length of which depends on the particular drugs used. Most leukemia chemotherapy is delivered intravenously and you may need to have a central venous catheter or port-a-cath (placed under the skin, in the chest), or a peripherally inserted central catheter (PICC line) inserted in your arm it more safely. This venous access device can also be used to draw your blood and to infuse fluids, antibiotics, and blood products should they be required. Some therapies are given by continuous infusion, either in the hospital or by a small infusion pump that you take home with you. Other chemotherapy agents can be injected subcutaneously or taken orally.

The chemotherapy enters the bloodstream and circulates throughout the body to attack and kill the leukemia cells. Chemotherapy is most effective in killing cells that divide rapidly. Leukemia cells are in this group, but so are some normal cells, especially those in the bone marrow, hair follicles, and those lining the gastrointestinal tract. That is why chemotherapy causes side effects related to reductions in RBCs (anemia), WBCs (infection), and platelets (bleeding); hair loss; and mouth sores, as well as nausea, and vomiting.

Each type of leukemia has different treatments and each of these regimens will be discussed in the next sections of this chapter. Chemotherapy is scheduled in cycles designed to maximize tumor kill while minimizing side effects. The number of cycles that you will be given depends on the type of leukemia that you have, the regimen chosen, and how you and your leukemia respond to the treatment. At the end of the chapter, an alphabetical list of the common chemotherapeutic agents, with a brief description of its particular characteristics, will be provided.

Potential Complications of Leukemia Chemotherapy

Tumor Lysis Syndrome. Since chemotherapy is designed to cause rapid killing of high numbers of tumor cells, it can lead to a complication called tumor lysis syndrome. This occurs when the leukemia cells break down and release their contents (including potassium, phosphate, and uric acid) into the circulation. High potassium levels in the blood can cause heart conduction abnormalities. Phosphates and uric acid can deposit crystals into and damage the kidneys. Zyloprim (allopurinol) is a medication that is prescribed before and during chemotherapy to help the kidneys excrete these cellular contents. You also will be given IV fluids with the chemotherapy and will need to make sure that you get enough oral fluids to help flush out the waste products of the destroyed cells. Lab tests will determine if any additional intervention is required.

Suppression of the Immune System

Infection. WBCs normally fight infection, but in leukemia most of the WBCs are abnormal tumor cells and are thus ineffective infection fighters. Infections are, therefore, quite common. Chemotherapy also contributes to this increased risk of infection, since it destroys normal WBCs inadvertently along with the leukemia cells. Specific symptoms of infection include cough, yellow or green sputum production, sore throat, painful urination, and diarrhea. In many cases, fever and chills may be the only sign of infection. When WBC counts are very low and the patient develops a fever, this is called febrile neutropenia and is a medical emergency. Intravenous antibiotics are generally needed to prevent complications and this may require admission to the hospital. When an infection develops in a patient with very few WBCs, they may not be able to mount a fever and may only have chills and shaking in response to it. This also must be addressed emergently as it may otherwise prove to be fatal.

RADIATION

Some patients with leukemia may require radiation therapy with their chemotherapy. This modality uses high-energy rays from a large machine. Rays are targeted to the diseased tissue by the radiation oncologist. In some patients, the radiation is directed at a specific region of the body where there is a large collection of leukemia cells, such as a lymph node mass or the spleen. Other patients receive radiation that is directed at the entire body (total body irradiation or TBI). This type of radiation may be used prior to a bone marrow/stem cell transplant. Radiation kills rapidly growing leukemia cells and does so at the point in their cell cycle when they are dividing. Therefore, it is best given in multiple sessions to affect the maximal numbers of cells.

BIOLOGIC THERAPY/IMMUNOTHERAPY

The use of natural substances, such as antibodies and cell growth factors, is called biologic therapy. These therapies can work by directly attacking the leukemia cells, as is the case with monoclonal antibody therapy, or by activating the patient's immune system to help fight the leukemia, which is the case with vaccines. Cell growth factors are called cytokines. They tell the bone marrow to produce specific types of cells.

Biologic therapies are effective in the treatment of many of the leukemias. Monoclonal antibodies may be used alone or in combination with chemotherapy and/or radiation. They are more targeted and will have less effect on the normal blood cells. They also have a different side effect profile. Antibodies are proteins that fit like a lock and key on antigens on the leukemia cells' surfaces. Once the antibody attaches to the cell, it brings in other immune cells to help kill the leukemia cells.

During initial treatments with monoclonal antibodies, infusion reactions may occur. These can be associated with fevers, chills, rash, fatigue, nausea, vomiting, diarrhea, difficulty breathing, and/or lowering of blood pressure. The reaction can be treated during and after the infusions with such agents as Tylenol (acetaminophen), Benadryl (diphenhydramine), and corticosteroids. The major risk with monoclonal antibody therapy is the development of infectious complications. Patients may require prophylactic antibiotics and antiviral medications to decrease this risk. Recovery of lymphocytes, and thus immunity, can take up to one year after completion of therapy. Other possible side effects include chest, abdominal, or back pain; mouth sores; loss of appetite; rash; itching; swelling; and blood pressure changes.

LEUKAPHERESIS

Leukapheresis is a process in which the patient's blood is passed through a special machine that temporarily removes the WBCs including leukemia cells and returns the remainder of the blood into the body. This is generally reserved for patients with extremely high WBC counts who cannot wait for chemotherapy to take effect.

SURGERY

Surgery plays less of a role in treating leukemia than it does in the treatment of solid tumors. Surgery may be performed to remove a lymph node for examination (biopsy). This is usually done to help make the diagnosis. Some patients with leukemia may also require surgical removal of their spleen, or a splenectomy. This is because the spleen is part of the immune system and acts by filtering blood cells. When a patient has one of the chronic leukemias, the spleen may become enlarged and uncomfortable, and create a risk for bleeding inside the abdomen. Large spleens can also trap normal cells, thus removing them from the circulation and causing blood counts to drop. Removing the spleen can help solve these problems. It can be done through an abdominal incision (known as an open procedure) or through a laparoscope (a minimally invasive procedure). The latter makes recovery easier for the patient.

BONE MARROW/STEM CELL TRANSPLANTATION

Some leukemias are best treated with bone marrow/ stem cell transplant. This is the most aggressive form of therapy for leukemia and is a complex procedure that requires a multidisciplinary team of physicians, nurses, social workers, pharmacists, and ancillary staff. It requires meticulous planning, and is typically done in tertiary centers. A detailed discussion on bone marrow/stem cell transplantation is provided later in this chapter (see page 53–57).

In both autologous and allogeneic transplants very high doses of chemotherapy are used to kill the leukemia cells. The dose of chemotherapy is so high that it also kills the normal bone marrow, or stem cells. The stem cells that are harvested from the patient (autologous) or donor (allogeneic) are used to rescue the patient's normal bone marrow by replanting it with stem cells so that it will function normally. Allogeneic transplant also produces an immunologic effect that works to kill the leukemia cells.

TREATMENTS SPECIFIC TO EACH
TYPE OF LEUKEMIA

CHRONIC LYMPHOCYTIC LEUKEMIA

Since the median age of CLL diagnosis is 72 years of age (though it has been diagnosed in those in their 20s), and the disease generally develops slowly, there may be few, or no, changes in the patient's health for many years. Many patients therefore never require any therapy for their disease.

Some people develop an enlarged lymph node, or multiple large nodal masses. Unless these are painful or are obstructing an organ, they will not generally require treatment. High WBC counts alone do not require therapy either, unless the bone marrow becomes so crowded that the RBCs and platelets drop to levels of concern in terms of the risk of anemia and bleeding. Other indicators that therapy is necessary include: otherwise unexplained fevers, night sweats, unintentional weight loss, frequent infections (especially respiratory, sinus, and skin), progressive fatigue, or feeling ill without another explanation.

Holding therapy until the above-mentioned symptoms emerge is called watchful waiting. Though it is difficult to be told that you have leukemia, in most cases of CLL it is better to delay treatment until symptoms develop. Depending on the rate of increase of the lymphocyte count, patients may be watched indefinitely and evaluated on a 3–6 month basis with physical examination and blood studies. The decision regarding the best time to begin therapy is often complicated. You and your doctor will likely discuss this on several occasions during the course of your monitoring. When treatment is required, doctors may recommend chemotherapy (orally, intravenously, or by catheter), radiation therapy, biologic therapy, or bone marrow/stem cell transplant.

Generally surgery is not used to treat CLL. One exception is when the spleen is involved and is causing symptoms such as pain, or is affecting RBCs or platelet counts. Radiation is also only used in special situations and does not play a major role in the treatment of CLL in most patients.

Treatment Goals

There is currently no cure for CLL, with the possible exception of bone marrow/stem cell transplantation. The transplant option is generally only considered for a small percentage of young patients with very aggressive disease as there is upfront mortality involved with the procedure as well as significant impact on quality of life. The goals of therapy for the majority of patients are to control symptoms, minimize infections, and to maintain a quality of life such that patients can preserve their level of functioning and continue to enjoy their daily activities. When chemotherapy or immunotherapy is used, normalization of counts and resolution of enlarged lymph nodes and/or spleen are additional goals. At present, it is also controversial whether a complete remission should be a goal or whether slowing the accumulation of CLL cells (partial remission) is good enough. This is, therefore, doctor and patient specific. Infection is often a big problem for people with CLL, so it is crucial to prevent and treat infections without delay.

Once treatment has been deemed necessary, there are many options that will be considered. Immunotherapy with or without chemotherapy may be proposed. Some of these agents may be given orally, or by a subcutaneous injection, however most of them are administered intravenously. They are often used in combinations.

Some of the decisions regarding which therapies to use are based on: the patient's age, other health problems, extent of involvement of the disease, and the results of the genetic studies, and surface markers of the CLL cells. Hematologists/oncologists generally have their own preferences for first-line therapy based on their experiences treating other patients. In CLL, there is a great deal of controversy regarding the best first-line therapy. In some respects, this is a positive sign in that it means that multiple therapies are effective.

Single agents that may be used include monoclonal antibody therapy alone—Campath (alemtuzumab) or Rituxan (rituximab) for first-line therapy. An oral alkalating drug called Leukeran may be prescribed with a corticosteroid drug called Deltasone (prednisone) for first line therapy as well. IV single agents include Fludara (fludarabine), Leustatin (cladribine), Treanda (bendamustine), Novantrone (mitoxantrone), and Nipent (pentostatin).

Combination regimens that may be used first line include: Fludara with Rituxan (FR), Fludara with Cytoxan (FC) and Rituxan (FCR), Fludara with Deltasone (prednisone) (FP), Treanda with Rituxan, Cytoxan with Oncovin (vincristine) and Deltasone. An alphabetized list of chemotherapeutic agents is included at the end of this chapter.

After the predetermined number of therapy cycles have been delivered, the therapeutic response will be assessed. Eradication of CLL cells from the blood and bone marrow, normalization of blood counts, and return of lymph nodes and enlarged spleens to normal dimensions means that the patient is in complete remission and may not need chemotherapy for a while (months to years). When the disease comes back, one or more of the above agents will be used in attempt to achieve another remission. Some of the agents are safer than others in terms of their effect on the bone marrow and organs. The hematologist/oncologist must account for these potential toxicities, monitor for them, and adjust regimens and dosages accordingly.

As is the case with the monoclonal antibodies, chemotherapy agents decrease the effectiveness of the immune system and increase the risk for infections. Some agents do so more reliably than others, therefore prophylactic (preventative) antibiotics are generally used with them to prevent infections that they are know to predispose to. For example, Fludara affects T lymphocyte function as well as that of the B lymphocytes. People with low T cells are prone to a type of pneumonia called *pneumocystis* pneumonia. A sulfa drug called Bactrim (trimethoprim-sulfa) is therefore prescribed with the Fludara-containing regimens to lessen this risk. Antiviral agents may be used to prevent shingles and antifungal agents may be used to prevent fungal lung, sinus, or skin infections.

Patients that require chemotherapy and/or immunotherapy for CLL are generally treated off and on for many years. As long as response continues and untoward effects are not interfering with quality of life, additional therapies will be offered. Since infection is the CLL patient's worse enemy, you must always monitor for fever and other signs of infection and report these to your treatment team immediately. Hospital admission may be required if you develop a fever when your WBC is very low. Hours of delay can make the difference between death and survival.

Ongoing Research

Fortunately, much research is being conducted to find better ways to treat CLL. Additional monoclonal antibodies, including humanized antibodies that may decrease infusion reactions, are now available while more targeted therapies are in development, as are CLL vaccines. Drugs used to treat other cancers are being used in CLL. One such agent is Revlimid (lenalidomide), an oral drug used to treat multiple myeloma. It is an immune system modulator that may stimulate a patient's immune system to attack the tumor cells.

The roles of many of the currently "experimental" agents are yet unknown. Many studies will be done to determine who will benefit most from each type of agent and what other agents they should be combined with.

Other Treatments

Radiation Therapy. Radiation may be used to treat CLL if there is a nodal mass that must be addressed rapidly, such as one obstructing the urinary tract or the gastrointestinal tract or one in any body region that causes significant pain. Otherwise its role in this disease is limited.

Surgery. A splenectomy (surgical removal of the spleen) may be warranted it if the spleen becomes very large and causes discomfort. Large spleens may also trap circulating RBCs and platelets and lower those counts to unsafe levels.

Treatment of Complications

Tumor Lysis. Tumor lysis syndrome and infection were discussed in the preceding sections (see page 31).

Transformation to a High-Grade Lymphoma. A major complication specific to CLL is that it can potentially transform into a more aggressive disease in a process known as Richter's transformation. After transformation, the disease is treated as a high-grade non-Hodgkin's lymphoma with regimens such as R-CHOP (**R**ituxan, **C**ytoxan, Adriamycin [**h**ydroxydaunorubicin], **O**ncovin, and Deltasone [**p**rednisone], which is given in 21-day cycles). The high-grade portion of the disease is potentially curable, however the low-grade portion (the CLL) will usually come back. Rarely, a CLL may transform into an acute prolymphocytic leukemia (PLL) that can be very difficult to treat. ALL may also develop, and would be treated as it would be in other ALL patients. AML is a rare complication that can result from damage to the DNA in blood-forming cells. This form of leukemia can also be very aggressive.

Hemolytic Anemia and Thrombocytopenia. In some cases, CLL can change the immune system in such a way that it begins to attack the patient's own RBCs (autoimmune hemolytic anemia) and/or platelets (immune thrombocytopenia). These conditions are initially treated with corticosteroids such as Deltasone or Decadron (dexamethasone). If these fail to work, or produce excessive side effects, intravenous immunoglobulin (IVIG), monoclonal antibody therapy (Rituxan) or immunosuppressive drugs may be used.

Recurrent Infections. The CLL itself increases risk of infection as it crowds out production of infection fighting cells. CLL therapies also decrease the functioning of the immune system as the immunoglobulins that carry around antibodies, and make them in response to infections, are destroyed by the CLL treatment. If immunoglobulin levels are low, especially if there is an increased incidence of infections, IVIGs may need to be administered.

Vaccinations, with the exception of live vaccines, should be administered as recommended (i.e., annual influenza vaccines, pneumococcal vaccines).

CHRONIC MYELOGENOUS LEUKEMIA

CML occurs mostly in adults with a median age at diagnosis of around 50 years. It affects approximately 1–2 individuals per 100,000. This disease is characterized by a specific genetic abnormality involving a switch in pieces of chromosomes 9 and 22 inside of the myeloid blood cells. The break on chromosome 22 involves a gene called BCR and the break on 9 involves a gene called ABL. When a piece of chromosome 9 attaches to the end of chromosome 22, the BCR-ABL cancer gene is made. It instructs cells to make the protein that leads to CML. Patients with this acquired genetic abnormality are said to have the Philadelphia Chromosome.

CML cells build up in the body over time, though some patients may not have any symptoms for a few years. The diagnosis may be made by an incidental finding on a routine blood test. One of the first indications of a problem may be a high WBC or platelet count, or a low RBC. If untreated, the CML cells eventually invade other parts of the body, including the spleen and can become a fast-growing leukemia (AML).

Fortunately, most patients are diagnosed in the chronic phase and there are excellent oral treatment options. If the WBCs that are affected are treated, the other cell lines are not affected and patients can return to their usual activities, though must remain on their medication for life.

In the accelerated phase, anemia develops and the platelets may also drop. WBCs can either increase or decrease in this phase. The patient may begin to feel ill as the numbers of blasts increase and the spleen begins to swell. This is the time that intravenous chemotherapy may be proposed.

When blast crisis occurs, the number of blasts is significantly increased in the peripheral circulation and in the blood. Patients feel tired and may be short of breath. They may also experience bone pain and abdominal pain. RBCs and platelet counts drop and there may be bleeding. Infectious complications occur as the WBCs present are not functional. A blast crisis signifies the transformation of CML to an acute leukemia (usually AML, but transformation to ALL also occurs). In all crises this transformation needs to be treated urgently as an acute leukemia.

Goals of Therapy

The goals of therapy during the chronic phase are to destroy all BCR-ABL gene-containing cells and to return the blood counts to normal. This should shrink the spleen and deter infections and unusual bleeding. This is classified as a remission in CML. In the accelerated and the blast phases, the goal is to return the disease to the chronic phase and to destroy all cells that contain the BCR-ABL gene.

During remission, patients feel well and can go about their activities normally, though this is not a cure. If treatment were to be discontinued for any reason, the disease would return.

Since 2001, CML has been treated with the oral agent Gleevec (imatinib) with much success. Prior to this, Roferon (interferon) was used to treat CML, and bone marrow/stem cell transplants were considered earlier in the course of the disease. Roferon was associated with a high rate of adverse effects such as causing patients to feel fatigued and achy a great deal of the time as if they had the flu.

Gleevec is an oral drug that targets the protein that makes CML cells multiply. It has drastically changed the way that

CML is treated and is now considered the standard of care. It may be the only agent that CML patients ever require. Gleevec is tolerated far better than its predecessor, Roferon. The most common adverse reactions include fluid retention, rash, muscle cramps, and diarrhea. These can be treated symptomatically. Other potential effects can include nausea, vomiting, bone pain, and lowering of any of the three cells lines. Many of Gleevec's side effects resolve after several weeks on the drug.

Tasigna (nilotinib) and Sprycel (dasatinib) are newer agents that are available for use if Gleevec stops working (drug resistance) or if the patient cannot tolerate it. These agents are also moving into the first-line treatment setting, as data is demonstrating efficacy and safety in patients who have not yet received any therapy.

Sprycel may cause lowering of counts, low calcium in the blood, changes in serum liver function studies, diarrhea, and headache. Tasigna's side effects are similar to those of Sprycel's and also include the potential for inflammation of the pancreas. In addition, Tasigna requires careful monitoring of the heart with electrocardiograms as it has been associated with abnormal rhythms that could cause dizziness or fainting.

Hydrea (hydroxyurea) is another agent sometimes used to treat CML, particularly when WBCs are extremely high. It is also an oral chemotherapeutic drug that suppresses the bone marrow and thus lowers all blood counts. This has to be carefully monitored and the drug titrated to the desired effect. Effects will last up to 10 days after the drug is stopped. Other side effects are rare and are reduced by dividing the daily dose and may include nausea, vomiting, mouth sores, rash, dry skin, and itching. Over time, this drug may produce permanent damage to the bone marrow and has been associated with the development of secondary malignancies (leukemia).

Other agents still occasionally used in the treatment of CML include Roferon-A with or without Ara-C (cytarabine), and Myleran (busulfan).

Leukapheresis

Leukapheresis (see page 33) may be considered if there are extremely high WBC or platelet counts that are causing symptoms such as those associated with blood clots or neurologic dysfunction.

Bone Marrow/Stem Cell Transplantation

Depending on the patient's age, performance status, overall health status, ability to find a matching donor, and response to the drug therapy, a bone marrow/stem cell transplant (see page 34) may be considered. Since the advent of Gleevec and the other similar agents, this is required far less often than in the past for patients with CML.

ACUTE LYMPHOCYTIC LEUKEMIA

Goals of Therapy

Patients with ALL must start therapy as soon as possible. The goal of therapy is cure—or at least a prolonged remission. Treatment decisions are based on: the number of ALL cells in the blood and bone marrow, analysis of chromosomes (those with certain chromosomal abnormalities fare better than do others), surface markers on ALL cells, age, and whether or not the leukemia has spread to the central nervous system (CNS). A remission in this disease includes return of blood counts to normal, relief of all disease-related symptoms, and killing as many ALL cells as possible.

Treatment

Treatment of ALL consists of three phases: induction, consolidation, and maintenance. Some drugs are given orally, while others are given through an intravenous catheter in the arm or upper chest.

Induction generally continues over a period of 8 weeks and consists of a combination of drugs that each work in a different way to kill leukemia cells. Current induction regimens for adult ALL combine Deltasone, Oncovin, and an anthracycline such as Daunomycin or Doxil (daunorubicin) with or without Elspar (L-asparaginase) and/or Cytoxan. Other agents that may be employed in ALL therapy include Clolar (clofarabine), Ara-C, MTX (methotrexate), Novantrone, Oncaspar (pegaspargase), and Decadron.

These agents, particularly in the dosage and combinations used, cause draumatic lowering of blood counts. During and after their use, patients are at increased risk from fungal, viral, and bacterial infections and cardiac toxicity is also possible. Nausea and vomiting are the most common gastrointestinal side effects.

Current multi-agent induction regimens result in complete response rates of approximately 74%–88% with a median duration of remission of approximately 15 months. You may also want to consider an investigational regimen. Ask your doctor if you are eligible to participate in a clinical research study. Information regarding clinical research is available on a number of the web-based resources listed in Chapter 11.

Supportive Care

Because of anticipated suppression of bone marrow as a consequence of both the leukemia and the treatment with chemotherapy, monitoring and supportive care are extremely important. The American Society of Clinical Oncology (ASCO) recommends that platelet transfusions be routinely given during induction treatment. Empiric broad-spectrum antibiotic therapy is often used and is crucial whenever fever (temperature greater than 100.5°F) develops in patients with low WBC counts. Hygiene is obviously very important. In rare instances, isolation and WBC transfusions may also be necessary.

The consolidation phase of ALL treatment follows induction therapy, but only if the induction treatment has resulted in a remission. If induction therapy has not produced a remission, it is repeated, either using the same regimen again or a different one. The definition of remission requires that each of the following criteria is met:

- Normal bone marrow (<5% blasts)

- No signs or symptoms of ALL

- No signs or symptoms of CNS or other organ involvement

- Normal lab values, including WBC count, differential, and platelet count

After patients have achieved remission, early consolidation therapy is used to prolong remission. It usually involves short-term intensive chemotherapy, followed by long-term maintenance therapy at lower doses.

Maintenance chemotherapy is the third and final phase of treatment. It follows consolidation chemotherapy, and usually involves 2–3 years of Purinethol (mercaptopurine) and MTX chemotherapy in an effort to prevent relapse of ALL. Deltasone and Oncovin may be added as well. Aggressive postremission chemotherapy in adults with ALL has shown a long-term, disease-free survival of up to approximately 45%.

CNS Prophylaxis

ALL cells may hide in the brain and spinal fluid and most intravenous chemotherapy does not readily cross into these areas. The use of prophylactic treatment of the CNS has greatly diminished recurrences, therefore early CNS prophylaxis is given to adult ALL patients during postremission therapy in an effort to prevent CNS relapse. Prophylaxis usually consists of intrathecal (directly into the spinal fluid) MTX and/or Ara-C and cranial irradiation. Intravenous high-dose MTX or Ara-C may also be administered. Radiation therapy may be administered to the brain or spinal canal to increase the efficacy of the chemotherapy in these areas.

Transplantation

Bone marrow/stem cell transplantation may be offered to patients who achieve an initial remission, though have a risk factor for relapse, such as in patients with certain chromosomal abnormalities. It is also indicated for relapse in bone marrow, brain, or testes after initial chemotherapy. Please refer to pages 53–57 for a more detailed explanation of the bone marrow/stem cell transplant process.

ACUTE MYLOGENEOUS LEUKEMIA

Treatment Goals

There have been tremendous advances in the treatment of AML over the past three decades and the percentage of patients attaining remission has increased significantly. Blood and bone marrow studies are conducted to diagnose the disease. They will reveal the cell type and demonstrate the characteristics of proteins on the cells' surfaces. Cytogenetic analysis is done to examine the chromosomes of the blast cells and together this information helps determine the best therapy for each patient with the disease. There are eight different subtypes of AML. Treatment can vary based on the subtype (Table 2). The subtype designation is based on the type of cell from which the leukemia developed as well as how mature the WBCs are. The classification is used to compare prognoses with certain subtypes deemed more favorable than others. M3, acute promyelocytic, has the most favorable prognosis. The M0 through M5 subtypes all start in precursors of WBCs, while M6 starts in early forms of RBCs. M7 starts in early forms of platelets. This can help explain some of the characteristic symptoms of the subtypes. For example patients with M3 AML, also known as promyelocytic leukemia (APL), are more likely to experience bleeding or clotting problems. It is important to accurately identify this subtype of AML to prevent these complications, and very importantly, APL is treated differently from most other forms of AML. It generally responds to vitamin A drugs, such as retinoids.

Besides subtype, other factors that imply that more intense chemotherapy is needed include: age (over 60 yrs), WBC count (over 100,000), history of former cancer requiring chemotherapy, certain chromosomal abnormalities,

Table 2 AML Subtype Designation

AML Subtype Designation	Cell Type	Special Treatment Considerations
M0	Undifferentiated myeloblastic	
M1	Undifferentiated myeloblastic, without maturation	
M2	Differentiated myeloblastic	
M3	Promyelocytic	Addition of all-trans retinoic acid (ATRA) to combination chemotherapy. Arsenic may be used.
M4	Myelomonocytic	Leukemia cells more likely to invade CSF. Patients require injections of chemotherapy into the spinal canal and may also need radiation if there is a large mass of cells in the brain or spine.
M5	Monoblastic	
M6	Erythroleukemia	
M7	Megakaryocytic	

certain gene deletions, and whether the AML developed from MDS.

Regardless of subtype, AML needs to be treated immediately. The mainstay of AML treatment is systematically administered combination chemotherapy that consists of two phases: induction to attain a remission and postremission consolidation therapy to maintain it. Induction with Daunomycin or Doxil and Ara-C is considered the standard combination therapy and is administered intravenously.

A minimum of 3–4 weeks on the inpatient unit is required. Adding other drugs together with this combination can increase the efficacy of treatment thus increasing the chance of remission.

Postremission consolidation therapy generally consists of one to four cycles of high-dose Ara-C containing regimens. This phase of treatment is also provided in the hospital and can take 3–4 weeks. Consolidation therapy may include either allogeneic or autologous bone marrow/stem cell transplantation.

Those with CNS disease will also require radiation to the brain and chemotherapy, as well as CNS treatment with MTX injected directly into the CNS. In AML, patients don't require prophylactic CNS treatment as do those with ALL, with the exception of the M4 subtype. Maintenance therapy has less value in AML; therefore, chemotherapy is not generally continued for more than 6 months after the initial remission has been achieved.

During the chemotherapy, patients may require RBC and/ or platelet transfusion support. Drops in WBCs last for a long time and can lead to infections requiring antibiotics until the counts recover. Growth factors may be used to increase WBCs. Other treatment-related side effects include rashes, dry mouth, mouth sores, nausea, vomiting, diarrhea, constipation, hair loss, and change in the taste of foods.

In addition the the chemotherapeutic regimen discussed previously, patients with certain AML subtypes may be offered the following "novel" agents:

> *Mylotarg.* Mylotarg (gemtuzumab ozogamicin) is a monoclonal antibody that targets CD33 myeloid cells. It is used to treat AML in older patients or in those

who have relapsed after, or are not strong enough to receive, chemotherapy. It is given by intravenous infusion after patients are premedicated to help prevent infusion reactions. These reactions generally occur during or up to 2 hours after the infusion and include low blood pressure, fever, chills, nausea, vomiting, hives, rash, fatigue, headache, diarrhea, and problems breathing. Neutrophils and platelets are the most commonly affected blood cells. Liver function studies may be transiently altered and patients may also develop nausea and vomiting as well as mouth sores not related to the actual infusion. Mylotarg is currently being tested in combination with chemotherapy in clinical trials.

Vesanoid. Vesanoid (tretinoin; all-trans-retinoic acid; ATRA) binds to protein within the cells and affects genes involved in the growth and proliferation of he leukemia cells. This agent is used to treat promyelocytic leukemia. There are also some effects on the immune system that are thought to play a role in fighting the disease. Side effects include vitamin A toxicity (headache [especially during first week of therapy], fever, dry skin and mucous membranes, swelling, mouth sores, rash, itching, and conjunctivitis). Abdominal pain is common and can be associated with either diarrhea or constipation. Cholesterol and triglycerides can increase, as can liver function tests, though this generally reverses when the drug is stopped. There may also be some CNS toxicity with symptoms such as numbness and tingling, imbalance, slow irregular speech, weakness, anxiety, or depression.

MYELODYSPLASTIC SYNDROME

Supportive Care

For some MDS patients, supportive care is the treatment of choice. The objectives are to maintain quality of life and minimize the need for frequent blood transfusions, minimize blasts, and delay progress to acute leukemia (including AML).

Subcutaneous growth factors may be useful and erythropoietin can increase RBCs in about 20%–40% of patients if these fail to elevate the hemoglobin to a safer and more comfortable level.

Growth factor injections for neutrophils (Neupogen [filgrastrim]), though not proven to be beneficial in terms of infectious complications, may improve the RBC response to the erythrocyte stimulating agents (Epogen [epoetin alfa]). If the growth factors do not provide an adequate response, transfusions are required for symptomatic anemias and antibiotics are administered for bacterial infections.

Agents Used to Treat MDS

When chemotherapy is necessary, the following agents may be considered:

> *Vidaza.* Vidaza (azacytidine) and Dacogen (decitabine) have been approved for the treatment of MDS and have been shown to decrease the need for transfusions as well as the risk for transformation of the disease into leukemia. Novel therapies such as Thalomid (thalidomide) have been used with improvement in anemia in about 1/5 of patients. These agents have side effects, the former myelosuppression, and the

latter nerve damage, fatigue, sedation and constipation. There are additional risks of dehydration, heart beat irregularities, infections, bone pain, and diarrhea.

Blood counts may worsen before they get better and supportive care may be needed, particularly in early therapy periods.

Revlimid. Revlimid is an oral drug similar to Thalomid that works by stimulating the immune system. It is, therefore, classified as an immunomodulatory agent. It is particularly effective for 5q minus MDS. Other actions of this drug that may contribute to its anti-cancer effects include inhibition of new blood vessel growth (anti-angiogenesis) and stimulation of normal programmed cell death (apoptosis).

The most common side effects include edema, itching, rash, constipation or diarrhea, nausea, joint pain, backache, cramps, dizziness, headache, insomnia, difficulty catching breath, fatigue, fever, and lowering of blood counts, especially in early treatment. Please also see the section on supportive care in Chapter 4. Supportive care plays a very important role in many of the leukemias and in MDS.

TRANSPLANTATION

Bone marrow/stem cell transplantation is offered to some leukemia patients to obtain a cure or to extend remission. Transplantation is an intensive treatment using very high doses of chemotherapy, with or without radiation, to kill the leukemia. In doing so, it destroys the bone marrow that then has to be replaced. When this intensive chemotherapy is given, it temporarily stops the patient from making enough blood and immune system cells. Stem cells are therefore harvested from the bone marrow of a suitable donor, usually a brother or sister (allogeneic transplant) or obtained directly from the patient (autologous transplant). A syngeneic transplant is marrow that comes from an identical twin, while a cord blood transplant involves the use of cells harvested from the placentas that are donated by mothers at the time of their baby's birth.

Regardless of the type of transplant, there are two ways in which stem cells are collected. One is by harvesting it from the posterior hip bone under general or spinal anesthesia. This generally takes 1–2 hours. The harvested marrow is processed to remove blood and bone fragments and a preservative is added so that the stem cell can be stored until it is needed.

Alternatively, stem cells can be obtained by apheresis. Since the goal is to obtain stem cells, and these do not normally circulate in the blood in large numbers, the donor must first be given small doses of chemotherapy and growth factors to mobilize the stem cells into the circulation. Apheresis involves placing an intravenous catheter and extracting blood, similar to the procedure used during blood donation. The blood then circulates through the machine that extracts the stem cells while the remainder of the WBCs, RBCs, and platelets are infused back into the donor through another catheter in the other arm. This process generally takes 4–6 hours.

After the patient receives the high dose induction chemotherapy (with or without TBI), the stem cells are infused, just like a blood transfusion, through the intravenous catheter. They then travel to the bone marrow and begin to engraft. Engraftment usually takes 2–4 weeks. Until it occurs, patients require intensive support with RBC transfusions, platelet transfusions, and growth factors for their WBCs. They also receive antibiotics and anti-viral drugs to prevent infections for 1–2 years, as it can take this long for the immune system to begin to work effectively again. The process of engrafting is monitored by frequent blood tests and marrow examinations.

Another option for allogeneic transplantation is a mini-transplant. This is a reduced-intensity or non-myeloablative transplant. This approach is currently being studied in clinical trials for various leukemias and lymphomas. It uses less toxic doses of preparative chemotherapy and/or radiation to kill some, but not all, of the patient's bone marrow, thus decreasing the number of leukemia cells. The donor cells, once they engraft, begin to destroy residual leukemia cells that were not killed by the chemotherapy given before the transplant. To boost this effect (also called graft-versus-tumor effect), the patient may be given an infusion of the donor's WBCs. Since the donor cells are not a perfect match, the donor's immune cells may recognize the patient's cells as foreign and attack and kill them. Some graft-versus-host effect is beneficial as the donor cells will attack any residual leukemia cells and hopefully prevent relapse. However, too much graft-versus-host can cause skin, gastrointestinal tract, and liver damage associated with sometimes disabling symptoms and fatal reactions. This is called graft-versus-host disease (GVHD). Patients require immunosuppressive drugs to prevent rejection of the donor marrow as well as to help prevent the development of severe GVHD.

Matching the stem cells with the patient's own stem cells as closely as possible helps to minimize potential side effects, particularly GVHD. Since people have different human leukocyte antigens (HLA) on the surface of their cells, potential donors are HLA-tested to determine how closely they match. This is done by a blood test prior to the transplant. Identical twins, of course, provide the closest possible match. Thereafter, close relatives, especially brothers and sisters, generally are the next best option. Each full sibling has about a 25% chance of providing an optimal match. The higher the number of matching HLAs, the greater the likelihood that the donor's stem cells will be accepted by the patient's body. Since only about 25%–35% of patients have an HLA-matched sibling, many patients require unrelated donors. When these are used, the matching potential is improved if patient and donor are from the same racial and ethnic backgrounds. Matched unrelated donor transplants are being increasingly used. Donors and patients should be in very good general health and there are age limit guidelines in various centers that are generally lower than those allowed for autologous transplants.

RISKS OF TRANSPLANTATION

In addition to the aforementioned risks of infection, bleeding, and graft-versus-host effects that occur during and immediately after the transplant, there are long-term risks as well. Infertility, early menopause, cataracts, and damage to the liver, kidneys, and heart are potential problems. These result from the pretransplant therapy, as well as that given during the transplant procedure itself. Specific side effects of each chemotherapeutic agent are discussed elsewhere in this and the next chapter.

Radiation, if given as part of the preparative regimen for the transplant, can cause inflammation of the skin and resultant discomfort. Damage to the lungs is called radiation-induced pneumonitis. It can produce shortness of breath and cough and this damage may be permanent. Liver related toxicity includes veno-oclusive disease (VOD) of the liver. This occurs in a small number and patients, and more so in those who have received TBI with chemo induction. VOD occurs early after induction therapy, and is associated with weight gain, edema, and jaundice, and may be fatal.

Late damage to the thyroid gland may occur, requiring thyroid supplements for life. Bone damage may occur and in extreme cases, parts of an affected bone or joint may need surgery for correction.

There is an upfront mortality risk involved with any bone marrow/stem cell transplant. It is estimated at 0%–5% for autologous transplants, and 10%–40% for allogeneic transplants. These statistics vary from patient to patient and each situation is different. The transplant doctors will discuss a more customized risk assessment after they have conducted a complete evaluation. Factors that alter risk include other diseases that you have going into the procedure, your age, and your performance status. Every attempt is made to screen for health problems that could increase the risk of death during the transplant period in an effort to best predict the risk for each patient. Infection is a major risk for all transplant patients.

CLINICAL TRIALS

Advances in the standard of care for cancer patients relies upon cancer patients participating in clinical research studies. In fact, many patients seek out the opportunity to participate in these clinical trials—particularly those in which the standard(s) of care have failed. There are likely to be trials for every stage of every type of leukemia.

You may not be interested in learning about the trials for which you are eligible. It is, however, the job of your doctors and nurses to inform you about them. Keep in mind that there are benefits to joining a trial and you owe it to yourself to learn what they are.

Some of these benefits include:

- Access to drugs or other therapies that are not yet approved for use in your disease and thus may be otherwise unavailable.

- The drugs being studied are often supplied free of charge by the companies sponsoring them.

- Strict protocols for symptom, lab, and radiology monitoring that provide another team of professionals responsible for your therapeutic progress are required.

- The opportunity to contribute to the scientific knowledge base that may positively impact other patients with your type of leukemia in the future, in addition to the potential to improve your own outcome.

Clinical trial participation is strictly voluntary. If you choose not to enroll in the trial that is offered, you will be offered treatment that is based on the current standards of care at your institution. If you enroll in a trial and change your mind at any time, you will be released from the trial and offered another therapy. You will also be released from a trial if your disease progresses while on the study, if you have side effects that cannot be managed successfully, or if your doctor determines that it is not in your best interest to continue for any other reason. The goal is for you and your disease to benefit from the therapy.

CHEMOTHERAPY AND IMMUNOTHERAPY DRUGS USED TO TREAT LEUKEMIA

A brief description of each chemotherapy agent follows (listed alphabetically).

Adriamycin (doxorubicin, hydroxydaunorubicin) is an anthracycline chemotherapeutic drug that is given intravenously as part of a multi-drug regimen such as CHOP. It is used more commonly in non-Hodgkin's lymphomas than in CLL and in most cases, is reserved for patients who have a conversion from CLL to a more aggressive lymphoma. It has cardiac toxicity so heart function needs to be monitored. There is a specified maximum cumulative dose (550 mg/m^2) that can be given to one patient (about 10 doses). It also has marrow suppressing qualities and affects the WBCs more than RBCs or platelets. Nausea and vomiting are seen, as are diarrhea, significant hair loss, and mouth sores. This drug can cause serious damage to blood vessels if it leaks out of the vein; therefore it is best given into a large vein through a port-a-cath or a PICC. It causes a red-orange discoloration of the urine 1–2 days after it is given.

Alvocidib (flavopiridol) is a drug that is being studied in clinical trials. It appears to be highly active in patients with high-risk genetic features of CLL and may work by preventing cells from progressing through their normal cell life stages, thus preventing them from proliferating. This drug is given by continuous IV infusion.

Ara-C is an antimetabolite chemotherapy agent that is used in several of the leukemias (including ALL). The major toxicity is lowering of the WBCs and the platelets. Nadir with this drug occurs between days 7 and 10. Lung toxicity has been reported with high-dose therapy with this drug. About 10% of patients develop nerve toxicity characterized by balance problems, lethargy, and confusion. This is generally mild and reversible and occurs most often in older patients. Redness of the skin can occur as can mild hair loss. This is one of the drugs that may be given directly into the spinal fluid. When given by this route, it may cause seizures, altered mental status, and fever within the first 24 hours.

Campath is a monoclonal antibody used to treat some forms of CLL. It targets CD52+ expressing lymphocytes. Antibodies are proteins that fit like a lock and key on antigens on the leukemia cells' surfaces. Once the antibody (in this case Campath) attaches to the cell, it brings in other immune cells to help kill the leukemia cells. The CD52+ antigen is on T lymphocytes as well as B cells, so this antibody can be used to treat T cell CLL as well as B-cell disease.

Campath can be given by an IV infusion over about 2 hours, or by an injection under the skin. It is given at a lower dose at first and gradually increased until the treatment dose (30 mg) is reached. It is then given 3 times per week for a total of 12 weeks. During early treatment with this agent, infusion reactions may occur. These can be associated with fevers, chills, rash, fatigue, nausea, vomiting, diarrhea, difficulty breathing, and/or lowering of blood pressure. The reaction can be treated during and after the infusions with such agents as Tylenol and Benadryl. The major risk associated with Campath therapy is the development of infectious complications. Patients require prophylactic antibiotics and antiviral medications to decrease this risk. Recovery of lymphocytes, and thus immunity, can take up to 1 year. Other possible side effects include chest, abdominal or back pain; mouth sores; loss of appetite; rash; itching; swelling; and blood pressure changes.

Clolar is an antimetabolite purine nucleoside analog used to treat ALL. This drug requires close monitoring for kidney and liver problems. Its major toxicity is lowering of blood counts. During and after its use, it puts patients at increased risk from fungal, viral, and bacterial infections. Cardiac toxicity is possible as well. Nausea and vomiting are the most common gastrointestinal side effects.

Cytoxan is an alkylating agent that is used to treat many leukemias and other cancers as well. In CLL, it is used in combination with other drugs and is a component of many of the multi-drug regimens (**C**VP, **C**HOP, **C**ytoxan–Fludara, etc). In ALL it may be used for induction therapy. It is generally given intravenously when part of a multi-drug regimen, though is available in an oral generic form. Its major toxicity is suppression of the marrow, causing drops in cell counts (most severely 7–14 days after it is administered—also termed the nadir of the counts); therefore the healthcare team will check weekly blood counts. This drug can be toxic to the kidneys and bladder and it is important to stay well hydrated to minimize these side effects (try to drink 3–4 liters of fluid per day). Ridges may occur in the fingernails and skin may darken slightly. These changes are temporary as is any hair loss that may occur

Dacogen is a hypomethylating agent used to treat MDS. In clinical studies it was given intravenously every 8 hours for 3 days (in 3-hour infusions) and repeated every 6 weeks. Blood counts may be decreased initially and other lab tests that may become abnormal include liver function studies, low sodium, high or low serum potassium, low serum protein, and low serum magnesium.

Decadron is a potent corticosteroid medication. It is used to potentiate some of the other chemotherapy drugs, but by itself can decrease lymphocyte counts. It also helps prevent nausea and rash and has potent anti-inflammatory properties. High doses are used to suppress the immune system in many autoimmune diseases. Even in lower doses, it can suppress the immune system enough to increase risk of infections. After long term usage, doses need to be tapered because the body gets used to not having to make its own steroids. It may increase hunger, fluid retention, and may disrupt sleep. Used long term, it can increase risk of infections, irritate the stomach lining enough to make it bleed, weaken the bones, and cause muscle wasting and cataracts.

Deltasone is a corticosteroid medication used in conjunction with other chemotherapeutic agents to augment their activity. By itself, it can kill lymphocytes and shrink lymph nodes, though generally not for prolonged periods. Long-term continuous use is associated with significant toxicities (bone loss, weight gain, swelling, cataracts, high blood sugar, and stomach ulcers). It is used in regimens such as CVP and CHOP for periods of 5 days in a row at the beginning of each 21-day cycle. It may cause some increase in appetite and energy as well as a disruption of sleep patterns. Corticosteroids also suppress the immune system functioning and may increase risk of certain infectious complications.

Doxil (doxorubicin liposome) is doxorubicin that is surrounded by a special covering made of a fat substance, called a liposome. This covering helps the drug survive the body's immune system so that it can go directly to the cancer. It is also given intravenously and may cause infusion reactions such as flushing or shortness of breath that can require treatment. It may lower blood counts and cause a condition known as hand-foot syndrome in which the palms and soles become red and painful and may peel or blister. This drug causes urine to turn red for 1–2 days after each dose and can cause damage to the heart muscle. It has also been associated with the development of secondary cancers. In general, side effects such as hair loss and decreased counts may be less than those experienced with the original forms of Adriamycin.

Elspar is an enzyme that destroys asparagines that the tumor cells need for the production of protein causing them to become rapidly depleted and die. This agent can be administered intravenously, intramuscularly, or subcutaneously. There is a risk of severe allergic reaction, but this is rare and can be prevented in most cases with antihistamine or corticosteroid premedication. It may also interfere with clotting of blood, may raise blood sugar, and can damage the liver. Since ammonia is a byproduct of asparagines, patients with liver dysfunction can experience elevated ammonia levels in their blood that could be toxic. The other common side effect is vomiting. Oncaspar is a modified version of Elspar.

Fludara is an antimetabolite chemotherapeutic drug from the purine analog class. Given intravenously, it can be used alone in CLL, or can be combined with other agents, such as Rituxan and/or Cytoxan, to enhance each agent's activity. Its main side effect is suppression of the WBCs, causing deceased lymphocytes, and an increased risk for opportunistic infections.

Prophylaxis with antibiotics and antivirals is thus generally advised. Fludara has also been associated with the development of hemolytic anemia in CLL patients, a condition in which the body attacks and destroys its own RBCs. In rare cases, aplastic anemia, or a decrease in all cell lines, has occurred. Nausea and vomiting may occur, but is usually very mild. Fever may occur from breakdown of tumor cells. Hair loss is generally not a major issue with this drug. Fludara is given the first week of a 28-day chemotherapy cycle for either 3, 4, or 5 days.

Gleevec is an oral drug that targets a protein that makes CML cells multiply. It has drastically changed the way that CML is treated and is now considered the standard of care. It may be the only agent that CML patients ever require. Gleevec is tolerated far better than was its predecessor, Roferon. The most common adverse reactions include fluid retention, rash, muscle cramps, and diarrhea which can all be treated symptomatically and may resolve after several weeks on the drug. Other potential effects can include nausea, vomiting, bone pain and lowering of any of the three cells lines.

Hydrea is another agent sometimes used to treat CML, particularly when WBCs are extremely high. It is also an oral chemotherapeutic drug in the antimetabolite category and its major effect is suppression of the bone marrow and thus lowering of blood counts. This has to be carefully monitored, and the drug titrated to the desired effect. Effects will last up to 10 days after the drug is stopped. Other side effects are rare and are reduced by dividing the daily dose. Over time, this drug may produce permanent damage to the bone marrow and possibly secondary malignancies.

Leukeran is an oral alkylating agent. It can suppress the blood counts for 4–6 weeks after a dose. It affects the white cells and the platelets more than the red cells. Long-term effects may include irreversible bone marrow suppression and increased risk of second malignancies including AML.

MTX is an antimetabolite drug that targets enzymes in the cancer cells to prevent them from moving through their cell cycle and by inhibiting their DNA synthesis and function. It is used for many types of cancers and has the ability to get into the brain and spinal fluid to treat any leukemia cells there when it is used intravenously. It can also be injected directly into the spinal fluid. Patients on MTX should not take supplements with folic acid as they can block its effect. They will likely be prescribed another form of folate (folinic acid also known as leucovorin) to take after the MTX to prevent its toxicities. The major toxicity is the lowering blood counts. Nadir occurs between days 4 and 7 and counts generally recover by day 14.

Mylotarg is a monoclonal antibody that is used to treat AML in older patients or in those who have relapsed after, or are not strong enough to receive, chemotherapy. It targets CD33 myeloid cells and is given by intravenous infusion. Reactions from the infusion may occur during or up to 2 hours after the infusion and include fever, fatigue, nausea, vomiting, rash, headaches, hives, low blood pressure, diarrhea, chills, and problems breathing. Neutrophils and platelets are the most commonly affected blood cells. Liver function studies may be transiently altered and patients may also develop nausea and vomiting as well as mouth sores not related to the actual infusion. Mylotarg is currently being tested in combination with chemo-therapy in clinical trials.

Novatrone is in the antitumor antibiotic class of chemotherapy drugs. It is given through an IV and may be combined with Fludara in the treatment of CLL, though is also used to treat AML. Cardiac function is monitored during treatment with this agent as it has been associated with decreased heart function, particularly in those with preexisting heart disease or hypertension, those previously treated with radiation or with anthracycline chemo drugs, and in the elderly. This drug can turn urine a blue-green color for up to 24 hours after it is administered.

Oncovin is a vinca alkaloid chemotherapy drug. It is given intravenously as part of a regimen such as CVP or CHOP. This agent may be associated with nerve toxicity over time, and may cause numbness and tingling of the fingers and toes. While many chemotherapy agents cause diarrhea, Oncovin causes constipation. It also causes hair loss, fever, rash, and mild marrow suppression and is damaging to tissues if it leaks from the vein.

Revlimid is an oral drug that works by stimulating the immune system. It is classified as an immu-nomodulatory agent. It is particularly effective for 5q minus MDS and is also being used to treat some CLL. Other actions of this drug that may contribute to its anti-cancer effects include inhibition of new blood vessel growth (anti-angiogenesis) and stimulation of cell death (apoptosis). The most common side effects include edema, itching, rash, constipation or diarrhea, nausea, joint pain, backache, cramps, dizziness, headache, insomnia, difficulty catching breath, fatigue, fever, and lowering of blood counts, especially in early treatment.

Rituxan is a monoclonal antibody that targets the CD20 antigen on B lymphocytes. It may be used alone or combined with other agents, such as Fludara and Cytoxan (FC) or Treanda in CLL. It is given intravenously and is associated with infusion reactions (fevers, chills, shaking, rash, hives, headache, breathing problems, nausea, and low blood pressure), particularly with the first and/or second dose. Subsequent infusions are generally easier. Suppression of lymphocytes is the goal, and its effect on other blood counts is rare but known to occur. It does not hurt the stem cells in the bone marrow, and mild nausea and vomiting may occur with subsequent infusions.

Tasigna and *Sprycel* may be used in CML if Gleevec stops working because of drug resistance or if you cannot tolerate it. Sprycel may cause lowering of blood cell counts, low calcium in the blood, changes in liver function studies (also in the blood), diarrhea, and headache. Tasigna's side effects are similar to those of Sprycel and also include the potential for inflammation of the pancreas. In addition, Tasigna requires careful monitoring of the heart with electro-cardiograms as it has been associated with abnormal rhythms that could cause dizziness or fainting.

Treanda is a newer chemotherapy agent for CLL that is administered intravenously over 30 minutes for two days in a row. This is done every 4 weeks and is dosed based on your body size. It is thought to work in two different ways: as an alkalating agent that causes DNA damage and as an antimetabolite that interferes with the production of new DNA. It may be associated with infusion reactions (fever, chills, rash), fatigue, diarrhea, and nausea/vomiting. It also may interact with other drugs that can affect its level its level in the body (Cypro [ciprofloxacin], Prilosec [omeprazole], Dilantin [phenytoin], Donnatal [phenobarbital], Luvox [fluvoxamine], Tagamet [cimetidine] and tobacco smoke). It is very important that your healthcare providers are aware of every drug that you are taking to help prevent you from experiencing toxic effects. Like most chemotherapy, this drug can lower blood counts and you will need close monitoring with blood tests. Other potential side effects include rash, fever, mouth sores, nausea, vomiting, and abnormal blood tests that could imply kidney or liver damage. When treating CLL, Treanda is generally administered with Rituxan.

VePesid (etoposide) is also called VP-16. It is a chemotherapy drug that is derived from a plant alkaloid and used to treat AML (also used in testicular cancer and small cell lung cancer). VePesid works by causing breaks in the DNA within the cells that causes them to die and is given intravenously, though there is an oral form of the drug. It may cause nausea and vomiting on the days that it is given, may cause some hair loss, lowers blood counts, and increases risk for infections as well as bleeding. VePesid may cause damage to nerves in the hands and feet called peripheral neuropathy, and the dose may need to be adjusted if this occurs. It is important to tell the treatment team if any numbness develops in your fingers or toes.

Vesanoid, used for some AML patients, binds to protein within the cells and affects genes involved in the growth and proliferation of the leukemia cell. There are also some effects on the immune system that are thought to play a role in fighting the disease. Side effects include vitamin A toxicity (headache especially during first week of therapy, fever, dry skin and mucous membranes, swelling, mouth sores, rash, itching, and conjunctivitis). Abdominal pain is common and can be associated with either diarrhea or constipation. Cholesterol and triglycerides can increase, as can liver function tests, though this is generally reverses when the drug is stopped. There may also be some CNS toxicity with symptoms such as numbness and tingling, imbalance, slow and irregular speech, weakness, anxiety, or depression.

Vidaza is a pyrimidine nucleoside analog agent that is used to treat MDS. It works by preventing a cellular process called methylation that shuts off the genes that control the development of cancer (the tumor suppressor genes). Vidaza is given by subcutaneous injection for 7 days every 4 weeks. The treatment goals are to reduce or eliminate blasts, improve RBC and platelet counts, and to delay time to development of AML. Potential side effects include chest pain, cough, fever, sore throat, skin redness, redness, pain and swelling at the injections site, rash, itching, bruising, constipation, diarrhea, nausea, vomiting, and loss of appetite. Joint pains may develop as may headaches, lethargy, and problems sleeping. Blood counts may worsen before they get better and supportive care may be needed during therapy, particularly in the early therapy period.

Please also see the section on supportive care in Chapter 4. Supportive care plays a very important role in many of the leukemias and in MDS.

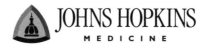

Be Prepared—
The Side Effects of
Treatment

L eukemia therapies have side effects. The type and extent of these will depend on several factors including the regimen used, your state of health going into treatment, your performance status, the type of leukemia that you have, and its stage or phase. Some of the most common side effects of chemotherapy are also common effects of leukemia itself, such as fatigue, anemia, low platelets, and increased risk of infection. In addition, some therapies affect people differently. While one patient may sail through a harsh regi-men of chemotherapy, another may experience disabling side effects from a therapy that is considered gentler. Fortunately, thanks to clinical studies, we have therapies for many of the side effects that you may experience. We will discuss some of the most common side effects here. Your doctors and nurses can give you guidance regarding what to expect in your particular case, and what can be done if you experience any unexpected side effects. Since these effects will also depend on the drugs that you are given, the dosage, and in what combination they are used with other agents. Your expected side effects will be discussed by your doctors and nurses in order to provide you with treatment modalities to hopefully prevent or minimize them. The specific side effect profile of the commonly used agents was discussed in detail in Chapter 3. In this chapter, we cover the more general side effects of leukemia therapy.

FATIGUE

Tiredness and fatigue is a common, almost universal, side effect of leukemia. The disease itself causes fatigue, as do most of the chemotherapy and radiation treatments. Patients describe this fatigue as different from the kind of fatigue or tiredness that they have been accustomed to experiencing in the past. Sometimes even the simplest tasks, such as getting dressed for an appointment, seem overwhelmingly difficult. Sleep may or may not improve this fatigue, but if it is part of the disease process, it should improve with treatment.

Anemia, caused by the disease or by the treatment, can be one cause of the fatigue, and blood transfusions may be required if the anemia becomes severe. Some patients may receive RBC growth factors such as Procrit (epoetin) or Aranesp (darbepoetin) to aid stimulation of the production of RBCs to help treat anemia and its related fatigue.

If you are ill for a period of time, and are not exercising and performing your normal activities for a while, it will cause you to become deconditioned and more tired. Many studies have shown that the proper amount of exercise is beneficial in both preventing and treating fatigue. Your healthcare team can advise you regarding safe levels and types of activities for you at the various stages of your therapy.

Sleep problems can also contribute to fatigue. If your sleep patterns become disrupted, there are sleep aids that your team may prescribe. Poor nutrition may be a factor as well, and you may be referred to a dietician or nutritionist if you are not able to eat a diet that provides adequate nutrients.

Whatever the cause, it is important to budget your energy and maintain realistic expectations. You will likely not be able to do everything that you did before your diagnosis, at least for some time. Prioritize tasks and perform the most important ones when you are feeling the strongest. Make a list of chores that need to be done and delegate to others. Even young children can help you conserve your energy by answering the phone when it rings so that you do not have to get up and walk across the room. Every little bit helps. There are other tips on the Web sites that are included at the end of this book.

PAIN

Pain can result from diagnostic procedures, infections, or side effects of chemotherapy and radiation therapy. Pain that you had prior to your diagnosis may become more problematic as you may be required to stop your previous medications during therapy. Many over-the-counter pain medications mask a fever that can be the first sign of infection and thus, you may be asked to stop taking them for a while. Alternative pain medications will be prescribed that do not mask fever and are safer for your liver and kidneys.

It is important to treat pain aggressively as it can severely impact your quality of life, contribute to depression, and prevent you from eating and sleeping well. Your mood, diet, and sleep are important to your overall well-being and ability to deal with the disease and its treatment. Pain interferes with every one of these aspects.

Don't be afraid to ask for and take pain medications if you need them. Though addiction is a major barrier to treating pain, it is extremely rare that a patient with cancer-related pain ever becomes addicted to pain medications. Your doctors and nurses can help you take pain medication safely, but it is your responsibility to let them know when you have pain, and how well their interventions relieve it. Pain is assessed on a scale from 0 (no pain at all) to 10 (worst pain you can imagine). You will become familiar with describing your pain's severity this way and it allows for much better pain management.

NAUSEA AND VOMITING

Nausea and vomiting are among the most feared side effects of cancer therapy. Fortunately they are generally preventable in most cases and treatable if they do occur. We now have excellent antinausea medications in pill form, intravenous form, rectal suppositories, and even in a skin patch form. Different chemotherapy regimens have different likelihoods of causing nausea, and you will be given treatment in the infusion center if you are receiving chemotherapy. You will also receive a prescription to take to your pharmacy, along with instructions on how and when to take the medications.

Your doctors and nurses need to know if you are experiencing nausea and/or vomiting. This is a very distressing symptom and can lead to dehydration quickly if not addressed right away. It is advisable to use some commonsense measures to help avoid these symptoms.

Temporarily altering your diet may help. Do not eat heavy or fatty meals before or immediately after a chemotherapy treatment. Avoid spicy foods. Make sure that you drink plenty of noncaffeinated beverages between meals. Try not to let your stomach get completely empty. Saltines may be helpful and peppermint and ginger candies may reduce queasiness as well.

INFECTION

Leukemia and its treatment both increase the risk of infection. When your immune system functions normally, it is capable of preventing many of the infections that you are exposed to on a daily basis. If a bacteria or virus does penetrate this defense system, another layer of your immune system attacks and kills the invading organisms. When your immune system does not work normally, it puts you at risk from infections that you are exposed to from others and your environment, as well as organisms that normally reside peacefully within your body.

Symptoms of infection include fever, chills, sweats, pain in the mouth or throat, cough (with or without mucous production), discharge from the nose and/or eyes, redness and pain in a joint or around a wound or incision, burning with urination, diarrhea, an area of unusual redness or swelling, change in mental status, and general malaise. If your immune system is compromised from chemotherapy and your WBC count is extremely low, you may have chills or shake but be unable to mount a fever. For this reason, when you become neutropenic, you may be placed on prophylactic antibiotics. If your WBC count is extremely low and you become ill, you may need to be admitted to the hospital for intravenous antibiotics.

Your temperature should be taken orally because rectal thermometer use could lead to dangerous infection and even bleeding when the blood counts are low. For this same reason, you are also asked to avoid suppositories and enemas when counts are low.

There are some commonsense strategies to help prevent infections that may arise from your environment. Stay away from obviously sick people. When your counts are low, avoid crowds, especially during cold and flu season. Avoid people who have received live vaccines. Don't garden or change cat litter in order to avoid exposure to bacteria or fungus in the dirt or litter. Some believe that you should also stay away from fresh flowers and live plants. Your healthcare team will let you know if and when this becomes necessary for you. Most importantly, wash your hands frequently and avoid touching your face in order to prevent the transmission of organisms to the mucous membranes of your eyes and mouth.

If you do develop any of the preceding symptoms, or a fever of or in excess of 100.5°F, you must notify the center any time, whether day or night. Early intervention can save your life, so keep their phone number handy.

MUCOSITIS

Mucositis is the medical term for mouth irritation or sores. It ranges from mild irritation to open ulcers and can actually occur anywhere in the gastrointestinal tract. Any opening in the mucous membranes is a way for infection to get into your bloodstream and this can be a serious issue when your WBC count is low. Chemotherapy kills rapidly growing cells such as those in the mucous membranes and therefore is a common cause of mucositis.

In leukemia and lymphoma treatment, steroids are frequently used as either a portion of the regimen and/or as premedication to prevent nausea and allergic reactions, as well as infusion reactions that may occur from the agents you are given. Unfortunately, steroids, as well as antibiotics, predispose you to fungal infections such as thrush. They can be treated with topical mouthwash that contains antifungal medication, lozenges, tablets, or, if severe, intravenous medication may be required.

If you have mouth irritation without thrush, you will be prescribed a special mouthwash that will coat the tissues and relieve the discomfort. Commercially available mouthwash products generally contain irritants such as alcohol and should be avoided. If mucositis becomes severe, pain medication is required in order for you to be able to eat and drink. Again it is crucial to advise your healthcare team so that this symptom can be effectively managed. You will also find it advisable to use a soft toothbrush very gently and to rinse your mouth frequently, especially after meals.

Regular dental visits and dental procedures are best done prior to your treatment if this is an option. Anything elective, such as crowns and cosmetic dentistry, should be put on hold during treatment. Consult with your leukemia care team prior to any dental work.

ALOPECIA (HAIR LOSS)

Therapies for acute leukemias and some chronic leukemias are likely to cause some degree of hair loss. Hair is another one of the body's rapidly growing tissues and is thus affected by chemotherapy. The amount of loss depends on the agents used and your healthcare team will tell you in advance what to expect. It generally begins shortly after the second cycle of chemotherapy is administered. Alopecia is less likely to occur during treatment for the chronic leukemias especially when only oral agents are used.

Hair loss is a distressing symptom for most people, women and men alike. Some prefer to buy a wig and most insurance companies will provide coverage for one. Others wear caps or pretty scarves. The American Cancer Society (ACS) has a wonderful program called Look Good, Feel Good that helps with this issue and offers information about how to use cosmetics to deal with the loss of eyebrows and eyelashes. Hair will grow back after therapy is completed. In the meantime, it is important to protect the scalp from the sun with a hat or other head covering, particularly when the weather is cold to help preserve your body heat.

CHEMO BRAIN (COGNITIVE DYSFUNCTION)

Chemo brain is a term used in the press as well as in the medical literature to describe problems with thinking and memory that can occur during and after chemotherapy. Little is known about the exact cause and course of this dysfunction and it is currently being studied. It is possible that some of this could be due to the stress of the illness, its effect on sleep patterns, and even some situational depression, in addition to any direct effect of the chemotherapy on the brain. Whatever the cause, this is a risk that is mentioned with many types of chemotherapy and is being taken seriously. If you notice changes in your ability to think clearly (fogginess) or seem to be forgetting things that were easy for you to remember in the past, bring this to the attention of your leukemia care team. It may be helpful to keep lists of things that you need to do and to keep a calendar to record your appointments and other activities.

CARDIAC CHANGES

There are several chemotherapy drugs that can cause damage to the heart including, but not limited to, Adriamycin and Cytoxan. Cardiomyopathy, or weakness of the heart muscle, can occur after chemotherapy treatments, but is not common. Heart failure can also occur but is rare, mild, and usually successfully treated. The key is close monitoring. To help evaluate your heart function and determine if it is safe and appropriate to give these medications, a special heart X-ray called a MUGA test is done prior to beginning therapy. Alternatively, an echocardiogram may be performed to assess the squeezing ability of your heart before you receive cardiotoxic chemotherapy, and may be repeated at certain points during your treatment. It is important to keep the treatment team apprised of any symptoms related to shortness of breath, cough, swelling, excessive fatigue, or chest pain.

NEUROPATHY

Some of the chemotherapies used to treat leukemia, such as Oncovin, are known to cause damage to nerves in the hands and feet. These peripheral nerves allow you to sense touch, pain, vibration, and temperature change. If they become dysfunctional, you are more prone to injury. The risk is greater if you have other conditions, such as diabetes, that can also damage your nerves.

The first symptoms are generally numbness and tingling that start at the tips of the fingers and toes and then progress up the hands and feet. This can turn into pain, and if the responsible drug is not stopped, the damage can be permanent and cause you to have problems buttoning shirts, writing, and perhaps even walking.

Part of your ongoing assessment involves questions about this symptom. Inform your care team when it starts so that they can monitor its progression in order to stop the agents or decrease the doses in time to prevent irreversible nerve damage. During and after therapy, if you develop nerve pain, there are agents that can be prescribed to lessen discomfort.

SEXUAL DYSFUNCTION

Loss of sexual desire is not uncommon during cancer treatment. Any of the aforementioned symptoms could obviously impact sexual function and can do so in both men and women. Whether it is due to the symptoms and therapy of the disease, or is stress-related, it is a problem that has not been fully studied. It is known that men may have difficulty sustaining an erection and may become sterile after treatment for acute leukemia. Women may fail to ovulate and may develop irregular periods, or even stop having periods altogether. Intercourse may become painful and extra lubricant may be required because of the disruption of the hormone levels. Other menopausal symptoms such as hot flashes, night sweats, irritability, and insomnia can contribute to a loss of interest in sex.

Intimacy is an important aspect of relationships and intercourse is only one way to demonstrate and receive affection. It is important to be open with your partner and explain your feelings.

There may be times during the course of therapy when you will be advised to abstain from sexual intercourse such as if your neutrophils or your platelets are dangerously low. Sexual activity could increase your risk for infection and bleeding.

In some cases, chemotherapy can affect one's ability to have children later. You will be informed if this a risk for you, based your plan of care. If so, you will be advised of your options.

MOOD DISORDERS

Anxiety and depression are very common problems during any serious illness. Anxiety is most likely to occur at the various disease milestones which include symptom onset, diagnosis, and times of routine follow-up evaluations. Unpleasant procedures and medications can also cause anxiety or make it more intense. Patients generally describe a sense of feeling ill at ease. They worry, become irritable, have problems sleeping, and may have changes in their eating patterns. Some patients develop a rapid heartbeat, palpitations, chest tightness, problems catching their breath, dizziness, difficulty swallowing, nausea, vomiting, diarrhea, and/or sweating. Anxiety can lead to panic disorder if not treated, in addition to making leukemia treatment much more difficult to tolerate. Treatment is available and may include individual or group therapy and perhaps medications

Depression includes prolonged feelings of sadness, hopelessness, helplessness, guilt, and inability to experience joy in formerly enjoyable activities. Everyone feels sad now and then, but if these symptoms last for more than 2 weeks, treatment for depression may be warranted. Depression and pain are closely related as depression can make pain feel worse and pain can cause depression if it lasts too long. If you are in pain, treating the pain is the first step. Depression can negatively impact sleep and nutrition and again, make life seem much more difficult than it would otherwise. Therapy and medications are readily available and should be initiated as soon as possible.

ANEMIA

Anemia is a common problem in leukemia and MDS. Although chronic anemia is not generally life threatening, it does impede quality of life due to its symptoms. The growth factors Procrit or Aranesp may be administered. These agents work by stimulating the bone marrow to make more RBCs, but this can take weeks to take effect. When Procrit is deemed appropriate, it may be given subcutaneously or intravenously. It is necessary to check your hemoglobin prior to each dose.

RBC transfusions may be required if the anemia is severe (hematocrit less than 25%), or if you are experiencing symptoms that could indicate that the anemia is affecting your heart or other organs. The frequency of transfusions will depend on your needs.

Risks of RBC transfusions include infusion reactions and accumulation of iron after repeated transfusions. This is a potentially dangerous condition, though there is effective treatment (iron-chelating drugs) to both treat and prevent it. Other risks involve the possibility of retaining too much fluid. You will be assessed for this when the doctors and nurses listen to your lungs before and after transfusions. Ankle swelling will be monitored as well as your weight. Diuretics such as Lasix (furosemide) may be given to help to eliminate the excess water in your blood stream. There is also a risk of transmission of viruses, though it is very small as the blood is carefully tested and donors are carefully screened. The most significant viruses that could be possibly transmitted include HIV, hepatitis B, and hepatitis C.

The risk versus benefit balance of blood transfusions generally leans in the direction of benefit when the hematocrit falls to 25% or less. You will be required to sign a consent form prior to receiving blood products. The risks will be discussed and your questions answered before you can receive blood.

NEUTROPENIA

When your WBC count is too low, you are at increased risk for infections. This can be especially problematic in patients with leukemia as the immune system is already compromised by the disease. Even a mild cold can turn into a life-threatening infection. WBCs cannot be transfused easily or safely in most cases. However, neutropenia may be treated with a granulocyte colony-stimulating growth factor like Neupogen, Neulasta (pegfilgrastim) or a granulocyte-macrophage colony-stimulating factor like Leukine (sargramostrim) that work by stimulating the bone marrow to make more infection-fighting WBCs. These are injected subcutaneously.

Antibiotic therapy is often used when neutrophils fall below 500. At this level, you are at risk from organisms that normally live in your intestines and do not cause you harm when your immune system is healthy. When you have too few neutrophils, bacteria may get into your blood and make you very ill. Prophylactic antibiotics may be used to prevent infection. When you are neutropenic, any fever that develops when your neutrophils are low must be treated immediately. Antiviral and antifungal drugs may also be used in either prophylactic or treatment doses.

When platelets are less than 10,000, there is a higher risk of bleeding. Because it can occur internally, it may not be as obvious as a nose bleed or bleeding gums. Bleeding can also occur under the skin and appear as bruises, rashes, or blood blisters. Rarely patients with low platelets don't see any bleeding, but develop headaches, increased weakness, or pain in the joints or muscles. Any bleeding, or suspicion of bleeding, must be immediately reported to the health-care team.

Bleeding prevention is extremely important in people with low platelet counts. Avoid playing contact sports, falling, and using dangerous equipment (such as electric saws), and shave with an electric razor instead of razor blades. Keep skin moist with lotions or creams to prevent cracking. Use soft-bristle toothbrushes to prevent trauma to the gums that could provoke bleeding. Keep stools soft to prevent straining from constipation and hard bowel movements. Diets with fiber from cereals, fruits, and nuts; sufficient fluids; and regular exercise will help. If this is not sufficient, use a stool softener and a mild laxative until the stools are soft enough to be passed easily. Inspect stools for blood, which indicates bleeding from the bowel or rectum, or dark tarry looking material which can indicate bleeding from the stomach. Check with your healthcare team before using rectal suppositories or enemas. They can be traumatic to the rectal tissue and create significant bleeding. If platelet counts fall too low, or there are any signs of bleeding, you may require platelet transfusions.

There are platelet growth factors that have been approved for other conditions. They are being studied in MDS and may be later used for leukemia patients as well.

SUPPORTIVE CARE

Supportive care is given before, during, and after treatment for leukemia. The goal of supportive care is to improve overall health and quality of life during the period that the chemotherapy or radiation is fighting the cancer, as well as after these therapies are no longer indicated. Supportive care can include dealing with the side effects of the cancer and its treatment as well as supporting nutritional and emotional health. Those with acute leukemia generally require more supportive care than do those with chronic leukemia. Some of the most severe effects of acute leukemia result from the bone marrow suppression that causes anemia, neutropenia, and thrombocytopenia. Many patients require transfusions of red cells and platelets during these periods. Treatment for bone marrow suppression is just as important as treatment for the leukemia itself, because having enough healthy blood cells will help you fight the leukemia better and survive longer.

EMOTIONAL SUPPORT

Supportive care also involves the mind and spirit. Don't let the leukemia control your life to the point that you have little or no enjoyment. Schedule plenty of time for fun, and spend time with family and friends. Go to a movie and have a good laugh. Play games that you enjoy and take frequent, even if short, vacations from the worry and stress of your disease and treatment. Balance is extremely important.

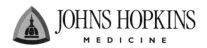

CHAPTER 5

STRAIGHT TALK— COMMUNICATIONS WITH FAMILY, FRIENDS, AND COWORKERS

Determining when and if to discuss your diagnosis and its implications with family, friends, and co-workers is often challenging. You need to decide how, when, and with whom to share this information. As the patient, all health-related information is yours, and you have the right to keep it private. However, depending on the type of leukemia, you may not have the luxury of complete privacy. For example, if your disease begins to cause weight loss, fatigue, enlarged lymph nodes, and pallor, or if you begin to lose your hair from chemotherapy, close associates will notice. You will likely require absences from work as well as disruptions in your other normal activities. This is difficult to hide indefinitely. Peoples' guesses about what is going on with you may be worse than the reality.

Some people feel the need to keep most of their personal information very private, while others need to share every detail. Some people withdraw from others during a crisis, while some rely on others readily. These characteristics are part of who you were when you started this journey, and leukemia is not likely to change this about you.

There are no right or wrong decisions. Think about the ramifications of your discussions and sharing of information. Use the resources that are available to you. Attending support groups and learning from others that have been in your shoes can be a tremendous help. Your doctors and nurses are likely to have opinions that are generally based on their interactions with patients that they have cared for throughout their careers. Listen to what they have to say as well. You may choose to enlist the support of a clinical social worker, psychologist, psychiatrist, or counselor. Do whatever it takes to feel comfortable with your communication "plan of action."

TELLING CLOSE RELATIVES AND SIGNIFICANT OTHERS

You may have been fortunate enough to have a spouse, sibling, or close friend with you through the evaluation process and at the time you learned about your diagnosis. If that is the case, this person can help you with the task of informing others. Most experts will tell you that it is important for you and your close relations that you share at least some basic information with them. As mentioned, people who are close to you will know when you are not well. If you hide facts, you are both depriving them of the opportunity to provide you with support that you need, and risking anger and hurt when they learn about the disease later.

It is common for different family members to have individual reactions to the diagnosis. Each person brings his or her past experiences with illness to the situation, along with their particular coping style and personality. Family crises tend to bring out either the best or the worst in each family member. Disagreements may arise regarding all aspects of the diagnosis, proposed treatment, and family plans that will need to be dealt with. Access to a good network that will provide support for everyone involved is important. Many families find social support from churches, spiritual groups, and community organizations. These resources should be tapped so that everyone feels supported throughout this difficult time. During these discussions, patients often begin to realize how much they mean to the others in their lives. One tactic is to just answer questions that are asked. That way, you are not providing unsolicited information. The process will likely be less scary for your family if they know the facts.

FRIENDS

Friends can be a tremendous support system when you are ill. They can provide a shoulder to cry on or help you laugh through some stressful times. During times of hospitalization and/or intense therapy, it can be of tremendous help if one person (preferably a natural born organizer) communicates the family's needs to the others in the larger social network. For example, friends can take turns making dinner for the family, driving carpools, etc. If someone else organizes this, you are not involved in the day-to-day conversations regarding arrangements. This is especially important for those of us who hate to ask for, or even accept, help from others.

Different friends serve different purposes in your life. Some you may share every detail and secret with, while others are those you enjoy on a more superficial level. Illness and therapy also differentiate types of friends. Some friends may be good listeners. Others may want to be directly involved with your treatments, such as providing transportation and/or sitting with you at the clinic. Others may not be able to handle anything to do with illness, but would be grateful for an opportunity to help by driving the kids to soccer practice. Tell friends what you want and need.

COWORKERS

As discussed earlier in the book, it is important to learn about your workplace's policy regarding absences and how flexible your schedule can be. It is a good idea to have a discussion with your supervisors so that you can assess their willingness to accommodate your treatments and periods during which you may not be able to work. Your Human Resources department may be able to help you decide what types of leave are available to you. Look into the Americans with Disabilities Act (ADA) for guidance. It is generally recommended that you complete the Family Medical Leave and Absence (FMLA) papers as early as possible. This, in essence, puts your employer on notice that you may require frequent visits for treatment and/or time off for hospitalizations.

Coworkers who care about you will also be curious as to what is going on. Use the guidelines that we discussed for close friends when deciding who to tell and how much to tell them. Generally they will be more willing to deal with the extra responsibilities that they may be asked to assume if they are in the loop.

TALKING TO YOUNG CHILDREN

Children need structure and a sense of consistency in their lives. They generally sense quite early when something is different in their home. Most experts believe that straight talk is best for them, and it is best if they get it from you. Children generally have fears that far exceed the reality of situations and reason to themselves that you are not telling them the truth because it is so horrible, not that you are trying to protect them. Deception may undermine their trust in you at a time when they need it the most. Every little detail is likely not necessary, but a general discussion regarding what is wrong (the level of detail may increase with age of child) and what you are planning to do about it is probably best. Answer the questions that they ask honestly, directly, realistically, and age appropriately. Don't be concerned about giving too much information. Children, like adults, will stop listening when they have heard enough. Providing information helps to correct any misperceptions about leukemia and its treatment. Understanding the importance of the treatment may help your child get through some difficult periods.

It is also important to remember that each child is different in terms of coping style, his or her preferences about the amount of information offered, and how he or she receives it. Provide each child the information that matches his/her ability to understand and process it. Allow children to process information in small amounts. You may need to provide it more than once. Older children are likely to want to know more about the illness and its treatment and have more sources to obtain information, including the Internet. Reinforce that all cancers and all people with cancer are different and that they should come to you if they learn or hear something that disturbs them. It may not be applicable in your case and they could worry for no reason. Encourage your child to talk about fears and concerns and admit that you are afraid and concerned as well.

Starting off with the acknowledgment that you have not been feeling well lately, such as by asking "I've been sick a lot lately, haven't I?", can help you determine what your child is thinking. Give your child outlets to express feelings. If you are spending a great deal of time in the cancer center, it is often helpful to let your child see where you are spending this time. If you are an inpatient, there may be restrictions about when and where on the unit they can see you. Your nurse can provide this information for you. Make sure that children know that someone (it is best to mention who, even if it is a long list of potential caregivers) will be there to take care of them so that they won't be afraid that they will be alone.

Let children know that your treatments may make you sicker before you get better, if this is the case. When you are experiencing side effects, let them know so that if you are less patient or become grumpy, they will understand that it is not their fault. Also let them know that leukemia is not contagious and that people close to you do not need to worry about catching the disease. Explain that there is nothing that anyone did to cause the cancer.

If you are comfortable doing so, inform your child's teachers about what is going on. They can then understand and deal with any sadness, tearfulness, distractibility, or behavior problems at school.

Children have amazing resources and capabilities. We can help to lessen some of the confusion they might experience by being truthful with them. There may be professionals available at your hospital or treatment center to help with your questions about how to talk with your children. The Leukemia and Lymphoma Society (LLS) can also direct you to resources and publications to assist you in communicating with your children. Again, social workers, counselors, and support groups can be tremendous resources in terms of relaying age-appropriate information to children. Ask for assistance in dealing with your child if he or she is having an especially difficult time dealing with the diagnosis, treatment, or post-treatment periods.

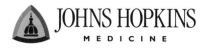

CHAPTER 6

JOHNS HOPKINS
M E D I C I N E

Maintaining Balance— Work and Life During Treatment

HOW TO PLAN CARE AND MINIMIZE DISRUPTIONS IN YOUR LIFE

You will likely need to cope with many changes and disruptions after your initial diagnosis of leukemia. The amount of disruption that will occur in your life will greatly depend on the type of leukemia that you have. Acute leukemias are the most disruptive as they must be treated urgently in most cases, and the therapy is prolonged and provided on the inpatient unit. On the other hand, some chronic leukemias will only require regularly scheduled clinic appointments. It is important to prepare for possible contingencies during any leukemia treatment. For example, infections with fever that occur during treatment may require emergent hospitalization for intravenous antibiotics. Some therapies must be delivered in an inpatient setting.

HOME LIFE

Try to maintain your children's routines as much as possible. They need to continue to go to school and to participate in sports and after-school activities as much as possible. Change creates stress no matter what the age. Plan ahead regarding who will take over for you in terms of childcare, carpools, meal preparations, and chores at home. Let them know in advance, if possible, when there will be an unavoidable change in their routines.

Keep children informed about what is happening related to treatment. Encourage them to help and play an active role in the treatment, too. If possible, allow them to visit the clinic to better understand what is happening and where you are spending your time. Have them draw pictures to cheer you up. They can open the get-well cards that you receive in the mail. Explain why you don't feel well and the importance of playing quietly on certain days after treatment. Let young children know that they can't catch leukemia and they also aren't the cause of it in any way either. Communicate with teachers, coaches, and counselors so that they are aware and can provide additional support.

If you are scheduled to have chemotherapy, make a chart of when your treatments will take place. Inquire about the possibility of having chemotherapy appointments toward the end of the week so you can have the weekend to rest up (when hopefully there will be additional help around the house available to you). Decide if you want someone to go with you for chemotherapy treatments. You may be in the chemotherapy infusion center for several hours, so plan accordingly. The day needs to be as laid back as possible for you. Depending on who is available to help and what your schedule looks like, you may decide the chemo days are pizza nights for the kids or to pull the casserole your neighbor made out of the freezer.

Children under stress may exhibit behavior problems. Though acting out is understandable, it should be addressed by setting limits. Show the child that his or her feelings are respected, though you still expect him to behave appropriately toward other people. Parents who ignore rules when the family is under stress have a more difficult time with their children when things get better. Consistent limits make children feel more secure and allow them to know what is expected of them.

Those who are close but outside the home will have expectations of you as well. This will start at diagnosis and continue throughout the treatment process. Family and friends will want to be kept posted on what is going on with you and your treatment. Consider group emails to provide a steady flow of information that will be released on your terms. This can prevent you from being bombarded with continuous phone calls and can be especially important during periods when you are not feeling your best.

WORKLIFE

At work, determine who needs to be notified if you are too ill to come in, or if you need to leave early for an appointment or test. Once you have a general understanding of what your therapy will entail, you can negotiate with your coworkers and decide on the best plan of action. For some, it will be necessary to take a prolonged leave of absence.

If it is possible to continue to work, determined by the disease and treatment schedule as well as how you feel, it is actually to your advantage to do so. Keeping your own life as normal as possible helps with coping and stress. It will also allow you to feel more productive, remain surrounded by coworkers, and have a distraction from your illness. Meet with your boss or supervisor and work out a schedule that works for both of you. There may be some days you only work half a day. Most bosses understand the importance of being flexible, and you are protected to some degree by the FMLA. If you work around small children though, especially toddler age, this may be problematic during chemotherapy since your risk of getting an infection is increased during this time.

WHEN YOU MIGHT EXPECT NOT TO FEEL WELL

Usually if you are going to have gastrointestinal side effects, it will be 16–48 hours after the infusion of the chemotherapy drugs. How you tolerate the first round of chemotherapy sets the stage for how the others using the same medicines will go. Request antinausea medications in advance so you can head off nausea and vomiting symptoms before they happen.

Fatigue caused by therapy generally progresses with each treatment. However, if your fatigue was disease-related, therapy may actually improve your stamina and endurance. Every case is different. Your healthcare team should be able to give you a general idea of what to expect.

INFECTION PREVENTION

There will be days when it will be anticipated that your WBC count will go down in response to having received chemotherapy. These are the days that you are more vulnerable to getting a cold, flu, or other form of infection. Eating a balanced diet rich in fruits and vegetables helps to improve your immune system. Washing your hands frequently is smart. Getting a flu shot before you start chemotherapy is advisable, too. Teeth cleaning and any dental work that needs to be done should happen before you start chemotherapy in order to prevent a problem related to tooth infections later. Chemotherapy doesn't cause dental problems but if one is brewing it can be made worse because your immune system is being taxed and is unable to fight infection as well as it did before.

If you need to travel by air while undergoing chemotherapy, and/or when your WBC count is low, wear a mask to reduce risk of exposure to the germs in the air that is recirculated on the plane. Your mission is to be as strong and healthy as possible during your chemotherapy treatments and to reduce the risk of exposure to infection as much as possible. The nurse working with you during your chemotherapy treatments can indicate on your treatment calendar the days that you will be particularly vulnerable to infection. Your blood will be periodically drawn to assess how your immune system is responding to the treatments and whether any medicines to boost your WBCs need to be administered.

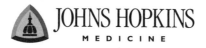

CHAPTER 7

SURVIVING LEUKEMIA— RE-ENGAGING IN MIND AND BODY HEALTH AFTER TREATMENT

SURVIVORSHIP

Taking an active role in your treatment and recovery may improve your quality of life during the period after treatment ends. One of the major goals of this book is to provide you with information based on facts and experience. Many people have friends and relatives who have known someone with leukemia. Cancer in some form is an almost universal experience in our society. Well-meaning folks will provide unsolicited information and advice. It is important to use appropriate filters and to not assume that these stories in any way mirror your circumstances. Rely on your healthcare team to help sort it out. They are the only people who are aware of and understand your particular circumstances, particularly your risk of recurrence.

No one can predict how you will respond to your treatment and you need to remember that your state of health, age, constitution, and personality will impact your experience. Survivorship is a period that offers unique challenges. During your post-therapy period, you will be assessed regularly with physical examinations, blood studies, radiologic studies, and perhaps bone marrow evaluations.

Returning to normal life after therapy means no more need for daily or weekly healthcare visits. The periods between assessments will lengthen the farther out from therapy that you get. One problem involves the expectations that you and others have regarding your ability to pick up your life where you left off. Readjustment can be as stressful and confusing as was the illness when you were first diagnosed. You may have changes in your appearance, energy level, stamina, and cognitive abilities to deal with. Some last longer than others and may in fact be permanent.

You will slowly transition back to your usual sources of health care for all non-leukemia related issues. At this point, your healthcare providers may not be as familiar with your disease and therapy. They also may not be aware of the long-term effects of the therapy. Survivors need to be their own advocates and be able to share this information with all future healthcare providers in order to receive the type and intensity of care that is required. It will help if you keep a record of your disease, its treatment, the dates of treatment, your schedule for follow up, and copies of all test results so that they are available for comparison.

LIVING A HEALTHIER LIFESTYLE

This is an excellent period during which to examine your lifestyle choices and make positive changes. Good nutrition can help you recover faster and stay healthier. Eat a balanced diet that includes plenty of vegetables, fruits, nuts, whole grain foods, and protein. Drink enough water and get enough restorative sleep.

If you smoke and have not quit, this would be a tremendous gift to give yourself and those who care about you. Quitting will improve your overall health, breathing, and sense of taste and smell. Examine how much alcohol you drank before your illness. Attempt to limit intake to one or two servings per day. Be sure to use alternative methods of stress control, such as exercise, relaxation techniques, and yoga.

Get an adequate amount of exercise. If you already exercise regularly, you can likely continue as long as you feel up to it. If you do not exercise regularly, ask your doctors or nurses about the best time to begin and how. Aerobic exercise, such as walking or playing tennis or basketball, can help strengthen your heart and lungs. Weight-bearing exercise can help strengthen bones and recondition muscles. Start slowly and listen to your body.

COUNSELING

The diagnosis of leukemia and the treatments required will undoubtedly be stressful for you and those who care about you. Take advantage of the counseling resources that are available to you. Your doctor will likely be able to recommend someone who is experienced in helping patients with the issues you are dealing with. Don't wait until you are feeling totally overwhelmed to ask for help. Alternatively, the hospital's social work department, the ACS, and the LLS can all be resources for you and your loved ones. Support groups are available in most areas and are extremely helpful.

LONG-TERM SIDE EFFECTS OF TREATMENT

Since becoming a leukemia survivor means that you have had leukemia, you will emerge from treatment as a different person in some respects. This may be a positive effect. Many cancer patients describe how their illness changed how they evaluate and prioritize issues and events, and helped them learn what is really important in their lives.

Since therapies are evolving and becoming increasingly effective, we will see more long-term survivors who may develop any of the potential long-term, or late effects, of leukemia therapy. It is therefore important to monitor for potential treatment-related effects that can occur months, or even years, after therapy is completed. The risk of development of a long-term effect may be affected by the patient's age at time of treatment, gender, overall level of health, and type and duration of therapy.

SECOND MALIGNANCY

The most notable long-term, and obviously most distressing, effect is the development of a secondary malignancy. Secondary malignancies are cancers that develop due to exposure to the chemotherapy and/or radiation therapy used to treat the primary cancer—in this case, leukemia. They may occur months to years later and are more common in those treated at a young age, and with higher total radiation or chemotherapy doses. Exposure to chemotherapy drugs including VePesid, Adriamycin, Blenoxane (bleomycin), Oncovin, Velban (vinblastine), Cytoxan, and corticosteroids have all been linked to secondary malignancies. The risk is thought to be higher if the patient received radiation therapy as well. High doses of alkylating agents, such as Cytoxan, have been implicated in the development of AML and MDS, as are high doses of VePesid. Radiation to the chest area, particularly in younger women, is a risk factor for the development of breast cancer later in life.

The most frequent type of secondary cancer is skin cancer, either basal cell or squamous. Fortunately these are slow-growing and easy to detect, treat, and cure. A yearly skin exam by a dermatologist is important for patients who currently have or have had leukemia.

When secondary cancers develop in other organs, they will produce symptoms specific to that organ. Be sure to report new or unusual symptoms to your doctors. In addition, maintain good preventive care practices and undergo recommended screenings such as mammograms, colonoscopies, and prostate checks.

PERIPHERAL NEUROPATHY

Damage to nerves in the hands and feet causes numbness, tingling, and even pain. This is called peripheral neuropathy and it may last for months or years after therapy with neurotoxic agents, such as Oncovin. There are some effective therapies for these symptoms and it is important to bring these symptoms to the attention of your healthcare team so that they will be provided to you.

HEART PROBLEMS

Potential damage from therapy includes heart failure and/or heart muscle injury that affects the ability of the heart muscle to squeeze well. This may occur shortly after, or years after, therapy with anthracyclines, such as Adriamycin, high doses of Cytoxan, or from radiation to the chest. The dose of anthracycline drugs is tracked so that it does not exceed the doses known to cause heart dysfunction. High doses of anthracyclines are used to treat AML. High-dose Cytoxan is used in the preconditioning regimen for bone marrow/ stem cell transplantation. The actual number of leukemia survivors who develop this late effect is quite small, but regular examinations are necessary. Echocardiograms or MUGA scans are used to assess heart function.

LUNG PROBLEMS

Lung tissue injury can occur from exposure to alkylating agents, from Blenoxane, and from radiation. Symptoms include cough, shortness of breath, and chest pain. If severe, emergent care is warranted. X-rays, CAT scans, and pulmonary function studies can be performed to confirm a problem and to follow responses to treatment.

COGNITIVE EFFECTS

Many survivors report changes in their thinking, focusing, and memory after treatment. Cancer therapy has been linked to a syndrome known as chemo brain (see Chapter 4) that can be associated with foggy thinking, disorientation, confusion, and the inability to focus on a task at hand or to remember things that were formerly easy to recall. This can range from mild to severe and must be differentiated from fatigue and depression, which cause these symptoms as well. Discuss this with your healthcare team, as there are some treatment modalities that can help, whatever the exact cause.

FATIGUE

Fatigue may not resolve completely in all patients, and it can last for months or possibly years. As the most common symptom experienced by cancer patients, it can interfere with activities of daily living. It can also be the most undertreated. There is a risk that fatigue may not be taken seriously by patients, family members, and even healthcare providers since it is not life-threatening. It can, however, be a major factor in preventing you from participating in and returning to the activities that you enjoy. Patients are told to expect acute fatigue during and after therapy. Most deal with a few weeks of fatigue and find this acceptable in terms of their treatment goals, especially if they involve potential cure. Prolonged fatigue becomes problematic in its effects on aspects of life.

Many factors have been found to be associated with prolonged fatigue including pain, fear, depression, sleep problems, anxiety, and ineffective breathing patterns. Symptoms that prevent adequate restorative sleep, especially pain, should be addressed. Sleeping medications may be required for brief periods of time in order to regulate sleeping patterns that may have been disrupted. Sleep apnea, which can be indicated by snoring and waking frequently during the night, requires specialized assessment and therapy. If fatigue is stable for some time and increases suddenly, it definitely requires a thorough evaluation.

Interventions to enhance restful sleep also include:

- Making the sleep environment sleep friendly. Darkness, quiet, comfort, and proper temperature are all important and white noise machines are helpful to some.

- Maintaining a sleep rhythm by going to bed and getting up at the same time each day.

- Curtailing time in bed to the time that you want to sleep and attempting to sleep only long enough to wake feeling refreshed. Avoid fragmented sleep as naps may not be helpful if they make you feel more tired and listless. They will also likely negatively impact your sleep at night.

- Avoiding food and drinks that could be stimulating (i.e., coffee, tea, or cola), especially after lunch.

- Avoiding alcohol before bed as this often causes fragmented sleep.

It has been demonstrated in many clinical studies that regular exercise improves fatigue. It helps to clear the mind; work the muscles, heart, and lungs; prevent blood clots; and enhances a sense of well-being. Start with light exercise and increase duration and intensity based on your endurance as well as your healthcare team's recommendations. Avoid temperature extremes when exercising and exercise the time of day when you are feeling the strongest.

Other tips for fighting fatigue include:

- Pacing yourself and prioritizing activities for each day. Less important activities can wait, or perhaps be delegated to others.

- Keeping a log of activities and exercising periods to help with planning ahead, as well as documenting your improvement. As fatigue lessens, gradually reintroduce additional normal activities into your daily routine.

- Eating nutritious, high protein meals and snacks throughout the day.

- Trying a bedtime snack to avoid hunger that could disturb sleep.

- Avoiding large quantities of fluids before bed because having to get up to use the bathroom is disruptive to sleep.

BONE DAMAGE

After treatment with chemotherapy and/or corticosteroids (such as Deltasone), osteopenia and osteoporosis, which is decreased bone density, may develop over time and will increase risk for fractures. There is also a risk of necrosis of the bone that can cause significant bone or joint pain. This is a condition in which the blood vessels that supply nourishment to the bone die, and the result is a weakening of that area of bone. There are surveillance tests and effective therapies for osteopenia. Osteonecrosis may require surgical treatment and any lasting pain in a bone or joint should be evaluated.

PREMATURE OVARIAN FAILURE— EARLY MENOPAUSE

Normal ovarian function can be suppresed by high-dose chemotherapy for leukemia, such as that given with a bone marrow/stem cell transplant. This can cause premature menopause and create fertility problems. These can be diagnosed by blood tests and sometimes treated with hormones. Bone strengthening medications, calcium, and vitamin D are given, because when ovaries do not produce estrogen, bones become weaker, increasing the risk for fractures.

No one can guarantee that ovarian function will not return. If you were treated prior to menopause, especially when in your 20s or 30s, there is a chance that your ovaries may begin to function again and your menstrual periods may resume. Thus, you should guard against the possibility of an unplanned pregnancy.

MALE STERILITY

In the case of men who have undergone acute leukemia therapy or high-dose chemotherapy, sterility may be temporary or permanent. Birth control should still be considered if the female partner is fertile until your healthcare providers inform you that conception is safe. It is important to allow enough time for all of the chemotherapy to be out of your system before risking a conception because chemotherapy drugs can cause serious birth defects.

THYROID DAMAGE

Damage to the thyroid gland from radiation therapy, such as that used in some transplant regimens, can leave it underactive. This is called hypothyroidism and may be associated with tiredness; sluggishness; changes in hair, skin, and nails; intolerance to cold; and changes in bowel habits. It can be detected with blood tests and treated with daily oral medications. Chemotherapy does not usually affect thyroid function.

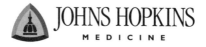

CHAPTER 8

MANAGING RISK—
WHAT IF MY CANCER
COMES BACK?

MONITORING FOR RECURRENCE

Worrying about the leukemia coming back is normal. It is one of the most common fears experienced after any cancer therapy. After therapy is given, you will be followed closely for an extended period of time. Your follow-up schedule will be determined based on the specific type of leukemia that you have, as well as the therapy that you received. The risk of relapse is different for each person, though your doctor may be able to give you some general guidelines regarding what to expect. You will be assessed at least once every 3 months for the first year.

Most doctors won't use the word cured when discussing results of leukemia therapy; the goal is to induce a remission. A complete remission, also called a complete response, simply means that no leukemia cells can be found on lab tests, in your bone marrow, or on scans. A partial response means that the disease partially responded to the treatment and is at least 50% reduced, though is still evident on tests. Stable disease means that the leukemia is not getting better, though is not getting any worse.

Keeping scheduled appointments and having all of the tests that have been ordered, and getting appropriate nutrition, exercise, and rest are all important in terms of your overall state of health. However, even if you follow all recommendations, the leukemia may come back. This may be because a small number of cells eluded the therapy and later began to regrow, or it may be because cellular DNA is damaged and mutates again as it did the first time.

You will be monitored for long-term effects of treatment (see Chapter 7) as well as recurrence of disease. During follow-up visits, your healthcare team will assess your blood counts and scans. You may require bone marrow examinations periodically as well. Specialized tests are required on a regular basis for some leukemias. For example, FISH and PCR will be done to assess for relapse of CML. You should alert your doctors in between visits if you develop symptoms such as fevers, frequent infections, enlarged lymph nodes, night sweats, spontaneous bleeding, excessive bruising, or unintentional weight loss. Remember that any of these symptoms is a nonspecific indication that something is going on, not a specific indication that you are experiencing a leukemia relapse.

If and when your disease recurs, doctors will address it as either a relapse or as a refractory disease. Relapse means that the disease recurred after having achieved a remission that lasted a reasonable period of time, such as 6 months. Disease is termed refractory when it stops responding to therapy currently being administered, or very shortly after therapy has ended. This means that the disease has become resistant to the therapy in much the same way that bacteria become resistant to antibiotics.

TREATMENT OPTIONS FOR RELAPSE OF LEUKEMIA

If your leukemia relapses, you may be offered another type of therapy. Your team may recommend chemotherapy, biologic therapy, or a bone marrow/stem cell transplant. This will be dependent on many factors, most importantly, the type of your leukemia and how it was treated initially.

ACUTE LYMPHOCYTIC LEUKEMIA

If ALL relapses after treatment, it may be treated with salvage therapy. This can involve retreatment with the initial regimen or high-dose Ara-C, MTX, or the hyper-CVAD regimen if the relapse occurs early after the completion of initial therapy. Clinical trials are being conducted to determine the effectiveness of monoclonal antibodies targeting leukemia-specific antigens that are attached to toxins or radionuclides. Allogeneic (donor cells) or autologous (own cells) bone marrow/stem cell tranplantation may also be used.

If ALL is Philadelphia chromosome-positive, Gleevec (the drug used in CML) may induce remission in some patients, at least for a short period during which a stem cell donor can be located.

ACUTE MYLOGENEOUS LEUKEMIA

Treatment for relapsed or refractory AML has to overcome drug resistance that likely occurred with initial therapy. High doses of Ara-C (HDAC), Novantrone, VePesid, MTX, or Fludara may provide short-lived remissions. Combinations of drugs may be used.

Other options include use of Temodar (temozolamide), which is an oral alkylating agent that is used for some brain tumors. It has been shown to have some activity against myeloid malignancies. Mylotarg has been approved by the Food and Drug Administration for targeted therapy in older patients who relapse after AML therapy. Transplantation still provides the best chance for a long, disease-free survival.

In patients who relapse after a transplant, conventional treatment options are limited, and enrollment in a clinical trial may be considered. Several targeted therapies are currently under investigation.

CHRONIC LYMPHOCYTIC LEUKEMIA

Since CLL is not generally a curable condition, it is expected to come back after remission. As mentioned, the goal is for a long remission, though some patients may have a recurrence shortly after chemotherapy has ended. Treatment options at this point depend on what the first-line therapy was and how long the remission lasted. If the remission lasted for years, sometimes doctors will reinstitute the same agent(s). Alternatively, drugs from different classes will be used in effort to achieve a second, third, or even fourth remission.

Though patients may have an excellent response to therapy and have their blood counts return to normal, there still may be very small numbers of leukemia cells in their blood, lymph nodes, or bone marrow. This is called minimal residual disease. It is not known whether it is necessary to continue treatment in asymptomatic patients until all evidence of disease is gone. Studies are being conducted to determine the answer to this question. Since CLL is not curable, some doctors believe that this additional treatment has more risks than benefits.

After prolonged therapy, the patient's major risk involves progressive negative impact on the immune system. Risk for infection increases and this poses the greatest threat. Prophylactic antibiotics may be instituted or reinstituted to minimize this impact.

CHRONIC MYLOGENEOUS LEUKEMIA

If CML progresses on Gleevec, one of the second generation agents can be used, and the other after that if necessary. Transplant then becomes the best option if your age and physical condition fit eligibility requirements. The potential benefits must outweigh the risks.

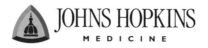

CHAPTER 9

My Cancer Isn't Curable—
What Now?

UNDERSTANDING GOALS OF TREATMENT FOR REFRACTORY DISEASE

Sometimes the leukemia keeps progressing despite being attacked by multiple forms of therapy. It may not always be possible to try another treatment, as the risk of additional treatment may outweigh any further potential benefits. At this point, the treatment may truly become worse than the disease.

Leukemia therapy is particularly hard on the bone marrow and may eventually cause it to stop working. Once the bone marrow fails, leukemia treatment is no longer possible. In this case situation, the disease makes the decision for us.

You may be offered additional experimental agents or clinical trials. After transplant, donor cells may be reinfused, or supportive care alone may be recommended.

The prospect of additional courses of therapy may simply not be something you want to pursue. You may have been told that you have a limited amount of time, and that anything gained from more treatment would be minimal. You may choose to live the rest of your life at home with family, doing things that you always wanted to do. This is a personal decision and there is never a right or wrong answer.

In either of the above scenarios, a transition between active treatment designed to attack the leukemia to one of control of symptoms, or palliation, is warranted. How you feel becomes the most important factor at this point.

QUALITY VERSUS QUANTITY OF LIFE

Quality of life is the focus in this stage of the disease. *Cure* is no longer an option, and *care* is the priority. The goal is to live the remaining time, whether it is days, weeks, or months, in comfort surrounded by those that you love, with dignity, and with your wishes respected. Having to get up, get dressed, and commute into the clinic or hospital is not the best option for care at this point. Instead, home care can be provided by traditional homecare nurses, or you can transition into hospice care.

HOSPICE/PALLIATIVE CARE

Comfort care, or palliative care, helps you feel as good as possible and manages any symptoms that develop. Palliative care treats symptoms, but is not aimed at controlling the disease. For example, radiation may be given to treat pain from an enlarged lymph node, though not with any intention of changing the course of the illness or prolonging life.

At some point, hospice care may be suggested. Hospice is a concept, not a place. Hospice care can be delivered in the home and focuses on comfort and family support. If you stay at home, nurses will come meet you and assess your needs. They are available for you 24 hours a day, 7 days a week and are the eyes and the ears of your doctors and cancer center nurses. A referral from your doctor is necessary and is usually made around the time the decision is made that treatment is no longer of benefit to you. Hospice nurses are experts at managing symptoms and improving your quality of life. They provide physical, emotional, and spiritual support—in keeping with your wishes—and will help insure a comfortable transition from quantity to quality of your remaining life. They have access to special equipment to help conserve your energy, and oxygen, pain medications, and medications to treat any symptoms that may develop along the way. They counsel family members who may be having as much, or more, trouble accepting the situation as you are. This is a very special time for most patients because you can spend your remaining time with loved ones. There are no more trips to the clinic and no more hospitalizations.

If home hospice becomes unrealistic because you need more care than your family can support, or your symptoms cannot be managed adequately anymore, inpatient hospice is available and follows the same philosophy in terms of comfort and surrounding you with family and friends.

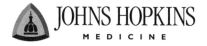

CHAPTER 10

JOHNS HOPKINS
M E D I C I N E

Leukemia in Older Adults

By Gary R. Shapiro, MD

L eukemia is a disease of aging. Contrary to what most people think, more older people develop and die from leukemia than do younger people. With the exception of the ALL subtype (which is usually found in young children and is quite rare in adults), the incidence of leukemia and MDS increases with age. Most diagnoses are made in men and women older than age 65. People older than 75 years have the highest rate of AML, and those in their 80s have twice the number of incidents of CML as those in their late 60s. CLL is the most common type of all of the leukemias, and its median age at diagnosis is 70. As we live longer, the number of people with leukemia and MDS will increase. In the next 25 years, the number of people who are 65 years of age and older will double, and the largest increases in cancer incidence will occur in those older than 80 years of age.

Older adults with cancer often have other chronic health problems and may be taking multiple medications that can affect their cancer treatment plan. Prejudice, misunderstanding, and limited access to clinical trials often prevent older patients from getting the timely cancer treatment that they need.

Older men and woman may not have adequate screening for leukemia, and when a cancer is found, it is too often ignored or undertreated. As a result, older individuals often have more advanced stage cancer and worse outcomes than younger patients. Older patients have less chemotherapy, less radiation therapy, and their leukemia is often left untreated.

WHY IS THERE MORE CANCER IN OLDER PEOPLE?

The organs in our body are made up of cells. Cells divide and multiply as the body needs them and cancer develops when cells in a part of the body grow out of control. The body has a number of ways to repair damaged control mechanisms, but as we get older, these do not work as well. Although our healthier lifestyles have allowed us to avoid death from infection, heart attack, and stroke, we may now live long enough for a cancer to develop. People who live longer have increased exposure to carcinogens in the environment from agricultural and industrial chemicals, drugs and chemotherapy, radiation, or certain viruses (see Chapter 1). Aging decreases the body's ability to protect us from these carcinogens and to repair cells that are damaged by these and other processes.

LEUKEMIA IS DIFFERENT IN OLDER PEOPLE

The biology of leukemia is different in older individuals than in younger people. Older patients with AML have a higher frequency of disease with genetic characteristics (multidrug-resistance phenotype and high-risk cytogenetic abnormalities) that are associated with resistance to treatment and poor outcomes. Preexisting myelodysplastic or myeloproliferative disorders are common in older patients, and AML that evolves from one of these is biologically more aggressive and resistant to treatment than other forms of AML. Indeed, older age is one of the most important poor prognostic factors, and a key indicator of survival in AML and CML. On the other hand, older patients with CLL tend to have more indolent disease than those who develop it when they are younger.

DECISION MAKING: 7 PRACTICAL STEPS

1. GET A DIAGNOSIS

No matter how "typical" the signs and symptoms, first impressions are sometimes wrong. That elevated WBC count or swollen lymph node in your neck may well be due to an infection or some other benign problem. Although enlarged lymph nodes may be a sign of CLL, other types of cancer often spread to lymph nodes, and their treatment and prognosis is usually quite different. Even when leukemia is diagnosed, it is critical that you and your doctors know what type of leukemia you are dealing with (see Chapter 1). For example, the acute types of leukemia (ALL and AML) can take your life quickly, and it is important to consider chemotherapy immediately. On the other hand, the chronic leukemias (CLL and CML) and most MDSs often have an extended period of slow growth that require less aggressive treatment than that which is used against AML. If you have CLL or certain types of MDS you may even live symptom-free for many years without the need for any anticancer treatment at all.

An accurate diagnosis helps you and your family understand what to expect and how to prepare for the future, even if you cannot get curative treatment. Knowing the diagnosis also helps your doctor treat your symptoms better. Many people find not knowing very hard, and are relieved when they finally have an explanation for their symptoms. Sometimes a frail patient is obviously dying, and diagnostic studies can be an additional burden. In such cases, it may be quite reasonable to focus on palliation without knowing the details of the diagnosis.

2. KNOW THE CANCER'S STAGE

Although the specific type of leukemia that you have is the most important factor in determining your prognosis and treatment options, knowing its stage is also quite important. No one can make informed decisions without it. Just as there may be times when the burdens of diagnostic studies are too great, it may also be appropriate to do without full staging in very frail, dying patients.

As discussed in Chapter 1, leukemias are staged differently than solid tumors. There are no standard staging systems for the acute leukemias, but disease status (untreated, remission, or recurrent), cytogenetic, and immunophenotypes are among the most important characteristics that determine treatment and prognosis in all patients with AML, regardless of age. As it is in younger patients, the stage of the MDSs and chronic leukemias (CML and CLL) is determined by careful examination of blood cells in the bone marrow and circulating blood. In CLL, the number and location of affected lymph nodes and the presence or absence of an enlarged liver or spleen are also important characteristics that can be assessed by physical examination and imaging studies. When doctors combine this information with information regarding your leukemia's subtype, they can predict what impact, if any, your leukemia is likely to have on your life expectancy and quality of life.

3. KNOW YOUR LIFE EXPECTANCY

Anticancer treatment should be contemplated if you are likely to live long enough to experience symptoms or premature death from leukemia. This will depend upon the type and stage of leukemia that you have, but it is almost always a consideration if you have AML or blast phase CML. If your life expectancy is so short that the cancer will not significantly affect it, there may be no reason to treat your cancer.

However, chronological age should not be the only thing that determines how your cancer should or should not be treated. Despite advanced age, people who are relatively well often have a life expectancy that is longer than their life expectancy with leukemia. The average 70-year-old woman is likely to live another 16 years, and the average 70-year-old man another 12 years. A similar 85-year-old can expect to live an additional 5 to 6 years, and remain independent for most of that time. Even an unhealthy 75-year-old man or woman will probably live 5 to 6 more years, long enough to suffer symptoms and early death from many forms of leukemia.

4. UNDERSTAND THE GOALS

The Goals of Treatment

It is important to be clear whether the goal of treatment is cure (induction and consolidation chemotherapy for acute leukemia) or palliation (chemotherapy for CLL, MDS, or resistant AML). If the goal is palliation, you need to understand if the treatment plan will extend your life, control your symptoms, or both. How likely is it to achieve these goals, and how long will you enjoy the benefits of palliation?

When the goal of treatment is palliation, chemotherapy should never be administered without defined endpoints and timelines. It should be clear to everyone what indicates success, how it will be determined (for example, by symptom control or improved blood counts), and when. You and your family should understand what your options are at each step, and how likely each is to meet your goals. If this is not clear, ask your doctor to explain it in words that you understand.

The Goals of the Patient

In addition to the traditional goals of tumor response, increased survival, and symptom control, older cancer patients often have goals related to quality of life. These may include having physical and intellectual independence, spending quality time with family, taking trips, staying out of the hospital, or even maintaining economic stability. At times, palliative care or hospice may meet these goals better than active anticancer treatment. In addition to the medical team, older patients often turn to family, friends, and clergy to help guide them.

5. DETERMINE IF YOU ARE FIT OR FRAIL

Deciding how to treat cancer in someone who is older requires a thorough understanding of his or her general health and social situation. Decisions about cancer treatment should never focus on age alone.

Age is Not a Number

Your actual age has limited influence on how cancer will respond to therapy or its prognosis. Biologic and other changes associated with aging are more reliable in estimating an individual's vigor, life expectancy, or the risk of treatment complications. These changes include malnutrition, depression, dementia, falls, and social isolation; and loss of muscle mass, strength, and the ability to accomplish daily activities such as dressing, bathing, eating, shopping, housekeeping, and managing one's finances or medication.

Chronic Illnesses

Older cancer patients are likely to have chronic illnesses (comorbidity) that affect their life expectancy; the more that you have, the greater the effect. This effect has very little impact on the behavior of the cancer itself, but studies do show that comorbidity has a major impact on treatment outcome and its side effects.

6. BALANCE BENEFITS AND HARMS

When one compares leukemias of similar type and risk profile, older patients with leukemia respond to treatment similarly to their younger counterparts. However, a word of caution is in order. Until recently, few studies included older individuals, and it may not be appropriate to apply these findings to the diverse group of older cancer patients.

The side effects of cancer treatment are never less severe in the elderly. In addition to the standard side effects, there are significant age-related toxicities to consider. Though most of these are more a function of frailty than chronological age, even the fittest senior cannot avoid the physical effects of aging. In addition to the changes in fat and muscle that you see in the mirror, there are age-related changes in your kidney, liver, and gastrointestinal function. These changes affect how your body absorbs and metabolizes anticancer drugs and other medicines. The average senior takes many different medicines (to control, for example, high blood pressure, high cholesterol, osteoporosis, diabetes, arthritis, etc.). This polypharmacy can cause undesirable side effects as the many drugs interact with each other and the anticancer medications.

7. GET INVOLVED

Healthcare providers and family members often underestimate the physical and mental abilities of older people and their willingness to face chronic and life-threatening conditions. Studies clearly show that older patients want detailed and easily understood information about potential treatments and alternatives. Patients and families may consider cancer untreatable in the aged, and as a result, may not understand the possibilities offered by treatment.

While patients with dementia pose a unique challenge, they are frequently capable of participating in goal setting and simple discussions about treatment side effects and logistics. Caring family members and friends are often able to share the patient's life story so that healthcare workers can work with them to make decisions consistent with the patient's values and desires. This of course is no substitute for a well thought out and properly executed living will or healthcare proxy.

While it is hard to face the possibility of life-threatening events at any age, it is always better to be prepared and to put your affairs in order. In addition to estate planning and wills, it is critical that you outline your wishes regarding medical care at the end of life, and make legal provisions for someone to make those decisions if you are unable to make them for yourself.

TREATING LEUKEMIA

YOU NEED A TEAM

Cancer care changes rapidly, and it is hard for the generalist to stay up to date, so referral to a specialist is essential. The needs of an older cancer patient often extend beyond the doctor's office and the traditional services provided by visiting nurses. These needs may include transportation, and nutritional, emotional, financial, physical, or spiritual support. When an older woman or man with leukemia is the primary caregiver for a frail or ill spouse, grandchildren, or other family members, special attention is necessary to provide for their needs as well. Older cancer patients cared for in geriatric oncology programs benefit from multidisciplinary teams of oncologists, geriatricians, psychiatrists, pharmacists, physiatrists, social workers, nurses, clergy, and dieticians, all working together as a team to identify and manage the stressors that can limit effective cancer treatment.

WATCHFUL WAITING

As discussed in Chapters 1 and 3, many men and women will carry a diagnosis of CLL or MDS that probably will not threaten their life spans. This is often the situation for older individuals who have a life expectancy of less than 10 years, or whose diagnostic work-up suggests low-risk disease. Some forms of CLL and MDS are detectable but never cause symptoms, while others grow progressively until symptoms appear. Although older men and women with chronic phase CML tend to progress to the blast phase faster than their younger counterparts, some will remain in chronic phase for 5 years or more. CLL and MDS are usually not curable, but most elderly patients' symptoms can be relieved with appropriate treatment so that they can live normal or near-normal lives for many years. Nearly three-quarters of fit seniors will live another 10 years after they are diagnosed with early stage CLL, and many will remain free of symptoms without treatment for quite a few more years. Although not many patients with advanced-stage CLL will survive more than a few years, treatment can often wait until symptoms appear.

High-risk forms of MDS, accelerated and blast phase CML, and all forms of AML are among the fastest growing forms of cancer. Symptoms usually develop in only a few weeks. If left untreated, these types of leukemia progress to death in only a matter of several weeks to months. Although these forms of leukemia are often resistant to treatment when they occur in older individuals, many seniors decide that the risks of chemotherapy are worth taking. Chemotherapy can be tough, but it is often the best way to control symptoms in all but the most frail man or woman.

CHEMOTHERAPY

Non-frail older cancer patients respond to chemotherapy similarly to their younger counterparts with leukemias. Though the side effects of cancer treatment are never less burdensome in the elderly, they can be managed by oncologists, especially geriatric oncologists, who work in teams with others who specialize in the care of the elderly. With appropriate care, healthy older men and women do just as well with chemotherapy as younger individuals. Advances in supportive care (antinausea medicines and blood cell growth factors) have significantly decreased the side effects of chemotherapy, and improved the safety and quality of life of older individuals with leukemia. Nonetheless, there is risk, especially if the patient is frail.

Myelodysplastic Syndromes

MDSs are a mixed group of disorders with a median age of diagnosis in the mid-70s. Some types of MDS can remain quiet for years, but others are characterized by progressive bone marrow dysfunction and the risk of transformation into AML. If the RBC counts drop low enough, the resultant anemia can cause symptoms like fatigue, angina, or shortness of breath. A low WBC count (leukopenia or neutropenia) can cause severe life-threatening infections, and thrombocytopenia may lead to bleeding. In the past, treatment of symptomatic MDS was limited to blood cell transfusions (RBCs and platelets) and antibiotics, but blood cell stimulating growth factors are now used to control complications of leukopenia (Neupogen, Neulasta, Leukine) and anemia. Revlimid (see Chapter 3) is a generally safe and well-tolerated palliative treatment for patients with transfusion-dependent anemia due to low-risk MDS, especially those associated with the deletion 5q chromosomal abnormality. Hypomethylating agents like Vidaza and Dacogen (see Chapter 3) may increase survival, decrease the risk of leukemia transformation, and improve quality of life (particularly fatigue and shortness of breath) in non-frail older patients with MDS. In addition to other treatment-related side effects, nausea, vomiting, and constipation may be problematic in frail older patients who are prone to dehydration and chronic bowel problems. Kidney failure, seizures, and heart rhythm disturbances such as atrial fibrillation may be more common in very elderly patients treated with Dacogen compared to those receiving Vidaza.

Chronic Lymphocytic Leukemia

Systemic therapy (see Chapter 3) should be considered for all but the frailest older patient with aggressive, symptomatic (e.g., profound fatigue, night sweats, weight loss, fever) advanced-stage CLL, especially those with related vital organ dysfunction, anemia, neutropenia, or thrombocytopenia. Oral Leukeran chemotherapy is effective and well tolerated in most older individuals. Intravenous Fludara chemotherapy probably yields more and longer lasting responses, but since patients treated with Leukeran live just as long, frail seniors should consider Fludara's increased toxicity before choosing it over Leukeran. Lowering the dose of Fludara does decrease the side effects, but the rate and duration of response is not that different than those of Leukeran. Although the addition of Rituxan to Fludara further increases the risk of toxicity, this chemo-immunotherapy combination does significantly increase response rates and survival. There are even more side effects with the Fludara, Cytoxan, and Rituxan (FCR) combination, but these can be managed and are no more common in fit older patients than in younger patients. FCR may be the most effective treatment regimen for symptomatic or high-risk CLL, and its use should not be based solely on chronological age.

Although Rituxan is usually given in combination with chemotherapy, as a single agent it may be a reasonable alternative for palliation in those too frail to tolerate one of the standard chemotherapy-based regimens. Even frail individuals have few side effects from Rituxan. Campath is a newer monoclonal antibody (immunotherapy) that is also well tolerated. It may be an excellent option for frail seniors or those who have had poor response to conventional first or second line regimens.

Corticosteroids (Deltasone or Decadron) can also be used to temporarily relieve symptoms in the frail elderly who are unable to tolerate aggressive chemotherapy, or for whom long-term survival is not a realistic goal. The presence of severe comorbidities, age-related frailty, or underlying severe psychosocial problems may be obstacles, even for these palliative treatment plans.

Chronic Mylogeneous Leukemia

Gleevec is as safe and effective in older as in younger patients. By and large, it has replaced Roferon, which is often poorly tolerated in the elderly, as the cornerstone of therapy.

Acute Leukemia

Intensive induction chemotherapy is often quite toxic in older individuals, even those who are quite fit. Nevertheless, it may be their only option for long-term survival or meaningful control of the symptoms due to acute leukemia. As previously discussed, acute leukemia in older patients is often biologically aggressive and resistant to treatment. Knowing the specific type and the genetic characteristics of an individual's leukemia helps identify those who have a chance of benefiting from this very aggressive therapy. Despite the risk of serious side effects, the fit elderly in this group generally do better with intensive induction and consolidation chemotherapy than a watch and wait approach or chemotherapy designed solely to decrease the number of WBCs. This cytoreductive approach uses drugs like oral Hydrea and subcutaneous Ara-C or Vidaza, and may provide some temporary relief from symptoms related to high WBC counts or those caused by anemia, thrombocytopenia, and neutropenia. This may be the best palliative option for unfit older patients and those with unfavorable biological profiles.

With regard to choice of chemotherapy, healthy older patients can receive regimens similar to their younger counterparts, including those that are anthracycline-based (see Chapter 3). Older patients are at increased risk of developing congestive heart failure from these regimens, and those with a significant cardiac risk need frequent monitoring, including serial echocardiograms. Unfortunately, when it comes to treating aggressive leukemias, there are no good substitutes for anthracyclines like Adriamycin. The less intensive anthracycline-free chemotherapy regimens may provide some symptom relief for those with aggressive leukemias, but they are usually less effective than anthracycline-based regimens. They should be reserved for patients with only the most severe cardiac disease.

TRANSPLANT

As discussed in Chapter 3, bone marrow/stem cell transplantation is sometimes used to treat CML, MDS, and acute leukemia, especially when AML or ALL is refractory to standard treatment. These are extremely risky procedures, even in the young and healthy. The risks increase dramatically with increasing age, and are usually over the top if you have any significant comorbidities. It used to be said that anyone over 50 years old should not have a transplant, but recent advances now make it possible for carefully selected fit seniors to consider these forms of aggressive therapy, especially the autologous type of transplant procedure. Although the risks of standard allogeneic transplant are usually too great for any older person, some transplant centers include the fit elderly in their mini transplants (nonmyeloablative bone marrow/stem cell transplants) research studies.

SURGERY

Surgery is usually not used to treat leukemia. However, a surgeon is often called upon to remove a lymph node so that a pathologist can determine if you have CLL or less commonly, some other form of leukemia involving a lymph node. This diagnostic biopsy is usually done as an outpatient under local anesthesia. It is a low-risk, routine procedure that is well tolerated by even those who are quite frail.

As discussed in Chapter 3, a splenectomy is sometimes recommended to treat symptomatic splenomegaly (enlarged spleen) due to CLL. It is as effective in elderly patients as in younger patients, but it does have a somewhat higher rate of complications in older individuals who have other medical problems. Like other treatment options, surgery in some older individuals may involve risks related to decreases in organ function (especially heart and lung), and it is essential that the surgeon and anesthetist work closely with your primary care physician or a consultant to fully assess and treat these problems before, during, and after the operation. Irradiating the spleen is a reasonable alternative for frail individuals, or for those with a very high surgical risk who are either refractory to systemic chemotherapy or too frail to get it.

RADIATION THERAPY

As in younger patients, radiation therapy provides excellent palliation in patients with CLL who have symptoms, like pain or obstruction, due to a mass of enlarged lymph nodes. It is particularly effective in treating pain. A short course of radiation therapy often allows these individuals to lower or even eliminate their dose of narcotic pain relievers. Although these medicines do an excellent job of controlling pain, they often cause confusion, falls, and constipation in older patients. Thus, even hospice patients suffering from localized pain or symptoms related to masses of malignant lymph nodes obstructing blood vessels, the gastrointestinal system, or the kidneys should consider the option of palliative radiation therapy for their CLL.

The fatigue that usually accompanies radiation therapy can be quite profound in the elderly, even those who are fit. Often the logistical details, like daily travel to the hospital for a 6-week course of treatment, are the hardest for older people. It is important that you discuss these potential problems with your family and social worker prior to starting radiation therapy.

COMMON TREATMENT COMPLICATIONS
IN THE ELDERLY

Anemia is common in the elderly, especially the frail elderly. It decreases the effectiveness of chemotherapy and often causes fatigue, falls, cognitive decline (i.e., dementia, disorientation, or confusion), and heart problems. Therefore, it is essential that anemia be recognized and corrected with RBC transfusions or the appropriate use of erythropoiesis-stimulating agents like Procrit or Aranesp.

Myelosuppression (low WBC count) is also common in older patients getting chemotherapy or radiation therapy. Older patients with myelosuppression develop life-threatening infections more often than younger patients, and they may need to be treated in the hospital for many days. The liberal use of granulopoietic growth factors (GM-CSF, G-CSF, Neupogen, and Neulasta) decreases the risk of infection, and makes it possible for older men and women to receive full doses of potentially curable chemotherapy.

Thrombocytopenia can cause serious bleeding problems. This is especially worrisome in an older person who is prone to falling. Someone who bleeds into the brain can suffer a serious and debilitating stroke. Like anemia and myelosuppression, thrombocytopenia is a side effect of many chemotherapy medicines and radiation therapy. It can usually be successfully managed by checking blood counts frequently and transfusing platelets when appropriate.

Mucositis and diarrhea can cause severe dehydration in older patients who often are already dehydrated due to inadequate fluid intake and diuretics (water pills for high blood pressure or heart failure). Careful monitoring and the liberal use of antidiarrheal agents, such as Imodium (loperamide), and oral and intravenous fluids are essential components of the management of older cancer patients.

Kidney function declines as we age. Some of the medicines that older patients take to treat both their cancer- and non-cancer related problems might make this worse. The dehydration that often accompanies cancer and its treatment can put additional stress on the kidneys. Fortunately, it is often possible to minimize these effects by carefully selecting and dosing appropriate drugs, managing polypharmacy, and preventing dehydration.

Neurotoxicity and chemo brain can be profoundly debilitating in patients who are already cognitively impaired (demented, disoriented, confused, etc.). Elderly patients with a history of falling, hearing loss, or peripheral neuropathy (for example, nerve damage from diabetes) have decreased energy, and are highly vulnerable to neurotoxic chemotherapy like Oncovin. Many of the medicines used to control nausea (antiemetics) or decrease the side effects of certain chemotherapeutic agents are also potential neurotoxins. These include Decadron, which can cause psychosis and agitation; Zantac (ranitidine), which can cause agitation; Benadryl; and some of the antiemetics, which can have a sedating effect.

Fatigue is a near universal complaint of older cancer patients. It is particularly a problem for those who are socially isolated or depend upon others to help them with activities of daily living. It is not necessarily related to depression, but can be. Depression is quite common in the elderly. In contrast to younger patients who often respond to a cancer diagnosis with anxiety, depression is the more common disorder in older cancer patients. With proper support and medical attention, many of these patients can safely receive anticancer treatment.

Heart problems increase with age, and it is no surprise that older cancers patients have an increased risk of cardiac complications, especially congestive heart failure, from anthracyclines, and other potentially cardiotoxic anticancer agents. Since it is such an effective drug in treating the acute leukemias, it is often used safely with careful monitoring in all but the most high-risk group of cardiac patients. Edema can be a problem in older CML patients treated with Gleevec. This can aggravate congestive heart failure in patients with heart problems; they need careful monitoring.

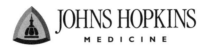

CHAPTER 11

JOHNS HOPKINS
MEDICINE

Trusted Resources—Finding Additional Information About Leukemia and its Treatment

Your healthcare provider is the best source of information for questions and concerns about your diagnosis and treatment. Because no two patients are alike, and recommendations can vary from one person to another depending on his or her personal circumstances, it is important to seek guidance from a provider who is familiar with your individual situation.

You can get reliable information from the following resources:

ORGANIZATIONS AND WEB SITES

American Cancer Society (ACS)
   (800) ACS-2345 (227-2345)
   http://www.cancer.org/

The ACS is a nationwide, community-based voluntary health organization and offers free booklets, programs, and support groups.

American Society of Hematology (ASH)

(212) 776-0544
http://www.hematology.org/
http://www.bloodthevitalconnection.org/
find-a-hematologist.aspx

Cancer Information Service of the National Cancer Institute (NCI)

(800) 4-CANCER (422-6237)
http://www.cancer.gov/cancertopics/types/leukemia
LiveHelp online chat: https://cissecure.nci.nih.gov/
livehelp/welcome.asp

The NCI offers comprehensive information about cancers and their diagnosis and treatment. It also provides current information about cancer prevention, detection, diagnosis, treatment, clinical trials, and rehabilitation, and helps with referrals for home care services and hospice.

Medicine Online

(714) 848-0444
http://www.medicineonline.com/topics/L/2/
Leukemia.html

Medicine Online offers information about diagnosis and treatment (including immunotherapy), with pages written by several physicians.

National Cancer Institute's Office of Cancer Survivorship (OCS)

http://www.cancercontrol.cancer.gov/ocs/
office-survivorship.html

The following is a list of related NCI materials and Web sites:

* *Chemotherapy and You: Support for People With Cancer*
  http://www.cancer.gov/cancertopics/
  chemotherapy-and-you

- Clinical Trials
  http://www.cancer.gov/cancertopics/factsheet/
  Information/clinical-trials

- Database of National Organizations That Offer
  Cancer-Related Services
  https://cissecure.nci.nih.gov/factsheet/
  FactSheetSearch8_1.aspx

- *Radiation Therapy and You: Support for People
  With Cancer*
  http://www.cancer.gov/cancertopics/
  radiation-therapy-and-you

- Taking Part in Cancer Treatment Research Studies
  http://www.cancer.gov/clinicaltrials/Taking-Part-in-
  Cancer-Treatment-Research-Studies

- *What You Need To Know™ About Hodgkin Lymphoma.*
  http://www.cancer.gov/cancertopics/wyntk/Hodgkin

- *What You Need To Know™ About Leukemia*
  http://www.cancer.gov/cancertopics/wyntk/leukemia

- *What You Need To Know™ About Multiple Myeloma*
  http://www.cancer.gov/cancertopics/wyntk/myeloma

- *What You Need To Know™ About Non-Hodgkin
  Lymphoma*
  http://www.cancer.gov/cancertopics/wyntk/
  non-Hodgkin-lymphoma

HELP WITH FINANCIAL OR LEGAL CONCERNS

Accompanying any serious illness are questions and concerns related to expenses incurred as a result of treatment, health insurance questions that can be overwhelming to try to understand or resolve alone, and sometimes even legal questions related to employment or financial matters.

The following is a list of national resources to aid you in addressing these types of concerns:

American Childhood Cancer Organization (ACCO)
(800) 366-CCCF (2223)
http://www.candlelighters.org
E-mail: staff@acco.org

ACCO offers support, education, and advocacy for children and adolescents with cancer, for survivors of childhood cancer and their families, and for the professionals who care for them.

Americans with Disabilities Act (ADA) Home Page
(800) 514-0301
http://www.ada.gov

Federal and state laws for Americans with disabilities protect qualified cancer survivors from job or insurance discrimination. The ADA Web site provides general ADA information and technical assistance materials. Publications can be downloaded through the Web site or ordered over the telephone. A free CD-ROM, which contains a collection of ADA materials, can also be ordered.

Employment discrimination is a potential problem for people who have had cancer. If you are one of 15 or more employees in your work space, you are protected against discrimination by this act and if you believe that your employer is discriminating against you because you used to be sick, you can contact the Equal Employment Opportunities Commission.

CancerCare, Inc.
(800) 813-HOPE (813-4673)
http://www.cancercare.org
E-mail: info@cancercare.org

Cancer*Care* is a national nonprofit organization that provides free, professional support services for anyone affected by cancer. This organization offers education, one-on-one counseling, financial assistance for nonmedical expenses, and referrals to community services.

Cancer.Net

(888) 651-3038
http://www.cancer.net/portal/site/patient
E-mail: contactus@cancer.net

The official patient information Web site of ASCO, Cancer.Net provides oncologist-approved information to help individuals and families make informed healthcare decisions.

CANCERVIVE, Inc.

http://www.cancervive.org
E-mail: cancervivr@aol.com

CANCERVIVE is dedicated to helping cancer survivors re-enter school or the workplace. It offers books and videos for adults, teens, and children; an "Ask the Expert" email for legal questions; and a listing of scholarships for cancer survivors.

The Cancer Legal Resource Center

(866) THE-CLRC (843-2572)
Email: CLRC@LLS.edu
http://www.cancerlegalresourcecenter.org

The Cancer Legal Resource Center is a joint program of the Disability Rights Legal Center and the Loyola Law School. It provides free and confidential information and resources to those with cancer-related legal issues.

Centers for Disease Control and Prevention (CDC) Cancer Survivorship Home

> 800-CDC-INFO (232-4636)
> http://www.cdc.gov/cancer/survivorship

CDC works with national, state, tribal, and local partners to create and implement successful strategies to help the millions of people in the United States who live with, through, and beyond cancer.

CureSearch

> (800) 458-6223
> http://www.curesearch.org

CureSearch represents the Children's Oncology Group (COG) and the National Childhood Cancer Foundation (NCCF). It supports lifesaving research, helps raise awareness of the importance of cancer clinical trials, and provides online information on types of childhood cancer and treatments.

Finding Cancer Support Groups in Your Community

> http://www.cancer.gov/cancertopics/factsheet/
> Support/resources

Job Accommodation Network (JAN)

> http://www.jan.wvu.edu/media/canc.htm

JAN provides free consulting services for individuals with physical or intellectual limitations that affect employment. Services include one-on-one consultation about job accommodation ideas, requesting and negotiating accommodations, and rights under the ADA and related laws. Although JAN does not help individuals find employment, JAN does provide information for job seekers.

The Lance Armstrong Foundation (LAF)

(866) 673-7205
http://www.livestrong.org/survivorcare

The LAF offers the LIVESTRONG Survivor Care program, which assists all cancer survivors. It provides practical information and tools; serves its mission through advocacy, public health, and research; and helps cancer survivors and family members face the everyday challenges of survivorship by offering emotional support, individual counseling, and assistance with financial, legal, and/or insurance issues and matching to clinical trials.

Learning Disabilities Association of America (LDA)

(412) 341-1515
http://www.ldanatl.org

The LDA was started by parents to offer other parents information on learning disabilities, tips on negotiating the special education process, and ways to help your child and yourself. The Web site includes an online training course about the Individuals With Disabilities Education Act (IDEA).

The Leukemia and Lymphoma Society (LLS)

(800) 955-4572
http://www.lls.org

The LLS is an organization with the goal of providing information and financial help to patients with leukemia. It also offers support groups for patients and families, provides referrals to other sources of help in the community, and supports cancer research.

Patient Advocate Foundation (PAF)

> (800) 532-5274
> http://www.patientadvocate.org

The PAF seeks to safeguard patients through effective mediation assuring access to care, maintenance of employment, and preservation of their financial stability.

Surviving and Moving Forward: The SAMFund for Young Adult Survivors of Cancer

> (866) 439-9365
> http://www.thesamfund.org

The SAMFund helps support young adult cancer survivors in the transition from high school to college and offers financial assistance through grants and scholarships.

The Ulman Cancer Fund for Young Adults

> (888) 393-FUND (393-3863)
> http://www.ulmanfund.org

The Ulman Cancer Fund for Young Adults addresses areas of cancer support, advocacy, and education for young adults dealing with cancer. It also connects young adults affected by cancer and offers financial assistance through grants and college scholarships.

BOOKS AND PAMPHLETS

What Is Cancer Anyway? Explaining Cancer to Children of All Ages, by Karen L. Carney

This book provides basic, reassuring information about cancer in simple terms. Published by Dragonfly Publishing, Inc.

The Jester Has Lost His Jingle, by David Saltzman

Written for children and teens, this story is about finding laughter and happiness inside oneself to help get through challenging times such as after a loved one is diagnosed with cancer. It is a useful tool for classroom presentations. Published by Jester Books.

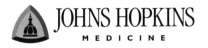

INFORMATION ABOUT JOHNS HOPKINS

Patients with leukemia are managed by the faculty of the Division of Hematologic Malignancies (as well as the multidisciplinary team that was described in Chapter 2) at the Sidney Kimmel Comprehensive Cancer Center at the Johns Hopkins Hospital.

Visit http://www.hopkinskimmelcancercenter.org/ for more information.

ABOUT JOHNS HOPKINS MEDICINE

Johns Hopkins Medicine unites physicians and scientists of the Johns Hopkins University School of Medicine with the organizations, health professionals, and facilities of the Johns Hopkins Health System. Its mission is to improve the health of the community and the world by setting the standard for excellence in medical education, research, and clinical care. Diverse and inclusive, Johns Hopkins Medicine has provided international leadership in the education of physicians and medical scientists in biomedical research and in the application of medical knowledge to sustain health since The Johns Hopkins Hospital first opened in 1889.

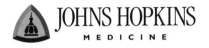

FURTHER READING

100 Questions & Answers About Leukemia, Second Edition, Edward D. Ball, MD, Jones and Bartlett Publishers, 2008.

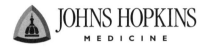

GLOSSARY

Acute granulocytic leukemia (AGL): This is a cancer of the blood in which too many granulocytes, a type of WBC, are produced in the bone marrow.

Allogeneic bone/marrow stem cell transplant: Stem cells collected from a donor and infused into the patient after high-dose chemotherapy.

Anemia: A condition in which the number of RBCs is less than normal.

Antibiotics: Drugs prescribed to treat infections, such as penicillin.

Apoptosis: Normal process by which the body replaces old or damaged cells with new healthy ones. Some cancer cells do not die, and a failure of cells to undergo apoptosis can contribute to the growth of cancer. Often referred to as programmed cell death.

Autologous bone marrow/stem cell transplant: Stem cells are collected from the patient and re-infused after high-dose chemotherapy.

B cell: Type of lymphocyte that fights viral infections and is important in immunity mediated by antibodies.

BCR-ABL cancer gene: A gene that has become mutated and tells the cell to make a protein that leads to CML.

Benzene: A chemical used to make plastics, pesticides, and detergents. Benzene has been linked to the development of some leukemias.

Beta-2-microglobulin: One protein on RBCs that is often used to assess both the extent of disease and prognosis.

Binet staging: Alternative staging system to the Rai system for CLL.

Bone marrow aspirate: A procedure in which a small quantity of marrow is removed via a needle placed through the bone and the cells are examined for diagnosis, staging, and assessment of leukemia and response to its treatment.

Bone marrow biopsy: A procedure in which a small piece of bone filled with marrow is collected with a special needle and the cells are examined for diagnosis, staging, and assessment of leukemia and response to its treatment.

Catheter: A tube inserted into the body to withdraw and/or deliver fluid or blood.

Central nervous system (CNS): The CNS is composed of the brain and spinal cord.

Chemotherapy: The use of chemical agents (drugs) to systemically treat cancer.

Clinical trial: A study of a drug or treatment to assess its efficacy and safety. Results are generally compared with those of the standard of care.

Complete blood count (CBC): Blood test used to assess numbers of RBCs, WBCs, and platelets.

Complete remission: No remaining evidence of leukemia on physical exam, X-rays, or laboratory tests.

Consolidation therapy: Treatment given after remission is achieved with the goal of killing any remaining leukemia cells.

Cytogenetic analysis: A lab test used to evaluative chromosomes in the tissue, blood, or bone marrow.

Cytogenetic remission: Post-therapy, there is no remaining evidence of leukemia in blood and/or marrow on cytogenetic tests.

Cytokines: Chemical messengers that are made by cells that act on other cells to increase or decrease their function.

Differential: An analysis of the percentages and absolute numbers of each type of WBC in the blood. This is generally ordered with the CBC.

Erythrocyte: A red blood cell.

Flow cytometry: A test in which fluorescent tags on cells' surfaces are counted to help diagnose type of leukemia and response to therapy.

Fluorescent in situ hybridization (FISH) test: Used to measure the presence of a gene or chromosome to help diagnose a leukemia and also to determine response to therapy.

Gene: The part of a cell that gives instructions regarding the making of proteins that help the cell perform its job.

Gleevec: Brand name for imatinib mesylate, which is in a class of drugs called tyrosine kinase inhibitors used to treat CML.

Graft-versus-host disease: GVHD is a condition that may occur after a bone marrow/stem cell transplant in which the donor cells attack the patient's cells, usually in the skin and the gastro-intestinal tract.

Hematocrit: The percentage of RBCs in the blood.

Hematologic response: Response to treatment in which signs of leukemia have resolved on blood tests.

Hematologist: A physician who specializes in disorders of the blood.

Hemoglobin: Protein in RBCs that carries oxygen.

HTLV-1: Virus associated with the development of some T-cell leukemias.

Immune system: Cells and organs in the body that protect it from invaders such as bacteria, viruses, and cancer.

Immunoglobulin: A protein in the blood made by B lymphocytes that helps the body fight infections. Gamma globulin is the most familiar immunoglobulin.

Immunophenotyping: A technique used to study the protein expressed by cells.

Immunotherapy: The use of immune cells to treat cancer.

Induction therapy: Initial treatment of cancer with chemotherapy or radiation therapy, with the hope of achieving remission.

Leukapheresis: Removal of WBCs by a special machine.

Long-term effects: Also called late effects, these side effects may occur months or years after completion of therapy.

Lymph nodes: Tissues in the lymphatic system that filter lymph fluid and help the immune system fight disease.

Lymphadenopathy: Enlargement of lymph nodes anywhere in the body which can be a sign of infection or lymphoma.

Lymphatic system: A collection of vessels with the principal functions of transporting digested fat from the intestine to the bloodstream, removing and destroying toxins from the tissues, and resisting the spread of disease throughout the body.

Lymphoblastic or lymphocytic: Type of leukemia in which the lymphocytes are the diseased cells.

Lymphocyte: A type of WBC that either produces antibodies to help fight infections (B lymphocytes), help the B lymphocytes make antibodies (T lymphocytes), or attack tumor cells and cells infected with a virus (natural killer cells).

Lymphocytosis: Elevated numbers of lymphocytes in the blood.

Marrow: A spongy substance within many of the bones in body.

Matched donor: Person with identical major tissue types.

Molecular response: Response to therapy in which no leukemia cells can be found by polymerase chain reaction.

Monoclonal antibody therapy: An immune therapy in which proteins are made to target a specific cell.

Monocyte: Type of WBC responsible for killing invading cells.

Myelodysplastic syndrome/myelodysplasia (MDS): Bone marrow disorder in which cells become abnormal and dysfunctional.

Myelogenous: The term describing the type of leukemia in which neutrophils are involved. Platelets and RBCs are also derived from the myeloid stem cell.

Neutropenia: A decrease in the number of neutrophils in the blood.

Neutrophil: Type of WBC that fights bacterial infections.

Nonmyeloablative bone marrow/stem cell transplant: Also known as a mini-transplant, an allogeneic bone marrow/stem cell transplant that does not use very high-dose chemotherapy.

Oncologist: A cancer specialist who diagnoses and treats malignancies.

Partial remission: A decrease in the size of a tumor, or in the extent of cancer in the body, in response to treatment. When you are in partial remission, between 50% and 99% of your disease is gone.

Pathologist: A specialist trained to distinguish normal from abnormal cells under a microscope.

Peripherally inserted central catheter (PICC): A long, flexible tube that is inserted into a peripheral vein, typically in the upper arm, and advanced until the catheter tip terminates in a large vein in the chest near the heart to obtain safer and more convenient intravenous access. Used for long-term infusion of bolus or continuous delivery of therapeutics or TPN drugs, fluids, nutrients, and chemotherapy.

Philadelphia chromosome: An abnormal minute chromosome found in WBCs in many myelogeous leukemias.

Polymerase chain reaction (PCR): Test used to detect numbers of leukemia cells that are below the levels that can be measured by cytogenetic methods

Plasma: The liquid component of blood containing proteins, hormones, natural chemicals, vitamins, and minerals.

Platelets: Small blood cells that prevent bleeding by forming clots at sites of injury.

Radiation therapy: Use of high-energy X-rays to kill cancer cells and shrink tumors.

Radioimmunotherapy: Treatment in which antibodies are combined with a radioactive substance and injected into the body to kill leukemia cells.

Radiologist: A physician specializing in the treatment of disease using radiation therapy.

Rai staging: Most common staging system for CLL in the United States.

Red blood cells: Cells in the blood whose primary function is to carry oxygen to tissues.

Refractory disease: Disease that fails to respond to any therapy or relapses within 6 months of chemotherapy administration.

Relapse: Recurrence of disease after it has been treated successfully.

Remission: A complete or partial positive response to therapy.

Risk factors: Any factors that contribute to an increased possibility of getting cancer.

Side effect: Unintended symptoms produced by a therapy.

Spleen: An organ of the immune and blood systems that is found in the left side of the upper abdomen.

Sprycel and Tasigna: Drugs used to treat CML after the patient becomes resistant to or cannot tolerate Gleevec.

Stem cell: Cell in the bone marrow that can become a WBC, RBC, or a platelet depending on the needs of the body at a particular time.

Subcutaneous: Located or placed under the skin.

T cell: Type of lymphocyte that is involved in cellular immunity and helps fight viral infections.

Thrombocyte: A platelet.

Thrombocytopenia: Too few platelets in the blood.

Vaccine therapy: Type of immune therapy for leukemia designed to increase the patient's immune system's ability to attack leukemia cells that persist after chemotherapy.

Watchful waiting: Common strategy in early-stage CLL. Physicians observe the leukemia with exams and periodic lab tests, though they do not treat the disease until symptoms emerge indicating that the RBC and platelets counts are falling below safe levels.

White blood cells: Responsible for fighting infections, total WBC counts are composed of lymphocytes, neutrophils, monocytes, eosinophils, and basophils.

INDEX

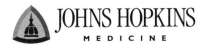

INDEX